Unifying Nursing Pr

Unifying Nursing Practice and Theory

Edited by

Judith Lathlean
BSc (Econ), MA

and

Barbara Vaughan
MSc, RGN, DipN, DANS, RNT

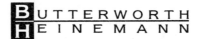

Butterworth-Heinemann Ltd
Linacre House, Jordan Hill, Oxford OX2 8DP

⟍Ⓡ A MEMBER OF THE REED ELSEVIER GROUP

OXFORD   LONDON   BOSTON
MUNICH   NEW DELHI   SINGAPORE   SYDNEY
TOKYO   TORONTO   WELLINGTON

First published 1994

RT73
.U614
1994

British Library Cataloguing in Publication Data
Lathlean, Judith
  Unifying Nursing Practice and Theory
  I. Title   II. Vaughan, Barbara
  610.73

ISBN 0 7506 1593 1

Library of Congress Cataloguing in Publication Data
Unifying nursing practice and theory/[edited by] Judith Lathlean and
  Barbara Vaughan.
  p. cm.
  Includes bibliographical references and index.
  ISBN 0 7506 1593 1
  1. Nursing – Study and teaching.   2. Nursing – Philosophy.
  3. Nursing – Research.   I. Lathlean, Judith.   II. Vaughan, Barbara, SRN.
  RT73.U614
  610.73'07–dc20
                                                              93–48048
                                                              CIP

Composition by R. H. Services, Hertford, Hertfordshire
Printed and bound by Biddles Ltd, Guildford and Kings Lynn.

Contents

Part Four   Alternative Approaches

Contributors

BURNS, Sarah   RGN, SCM, DN(Lond), DNE(Lond), BA
Lecturer Practitioner, John Radcliffe Hospital and School of Health Care Studies, Oxford Brookes University, Oxford, UNITED KINGDOM

COX, Helen   RN, DipNED(CNA), BAp.Sc(Lincoln Inst), MNS (LaTrobe), FRCNA
Senior Lecturer, School of Nursing, Deakin University, Geelong, Victoria, AUSTRALIA

FITZGERALD, Mary   MN, RGN, DN(Lond), CertEd(FE)
Post-graduate Student, School of Health, The University of New England, Armidale, New South Wales, AUSTRALIA

HANNA, Barbara   RN, RM, IWC, BNurs(Hons)
Lecturer in Nursing, School of Nursing, Deakin University, Geelong, Victoria, AUSTRALIA

HESLOP, Angela   RGN, RCNT, DN(Lond)
Senior Nurse, Nursing Development Unit and Respiratory Health Worker, Charing Cross Hospital, London, UNITED KINGDOM

LATHLEAN, Judith   BSc(Econ), MA
Professor of Education in Nursing and Director, GNC Trust Nurse Education Research Unit, Department of Educational Studies, University of Surrey, Guildford, UNITED KINGDOM

MACLEOD, Martha   RN, BA, MA, PhD
Project Adviser Nursing, St Boniface General Hospital, Winnipeg, Manitoba, CANADA

PEART, Kerry   RN, BNurs
Lecturer in Nursing, School of Nursing, Deakin University and Charge

Nurse, Professorial Unit, The Geelong Hospital, Geelong, Victoria, AUSTRALIA

SPARROW, Shelagh   MA, DN(Lond), RGN
Lecturer Practitioner in Research, Bloomsbury and Islington Health Authority, London, UNITED KINGDOM

STEVENS, Ingrid   MSc, RGN, RCNT, Royal Marsden Oncological Nursing Certificate
Lecturer Practitioner, Churchill Hospital and School of Health Care Studies, Oxford Brookes University, Oxford, UNITED KINGDOM

VAUGHAN, Barbara   MSc, RGN, DipN, DANS, RNT
Programme Director for Nursing Development, King's Fund Centre, London, UNITED KINGDOM

WRIGHT, Steve   RGN, DN(Lond), RCNT, DANS, RNT, MSc
Director, The European Nursing Development Agency, Tameside, Lancashire, UNITED KINGDOM

Introduction

The origins of this book lie in a deep-seated concern by all those who have contributed to it about the widening gaps which have arisen in the past between nursing practice, education, research and management. It would be unrealistic and indeed undesirable to expect an exact fit between espoused and used theory. Nor would it be desirable to find a total consensus about nursing theory. In either of these situations there would be no room left for growth and development. However neither is it acceptable to generate situations which do not allow an interface for dialogue between those who practice and those whose prime interest is education, research or management.

The current position has been enhanced by major changes in nurse education over the past decade. A significant amount of research has been undertaken in this area, particularly examining clinical learning environments as well as the difficulties experienced in the use of research-based knowledge in practice. Recently attempts have been made, influenced in part by the advent of the changes in initial nurse education but also by a growing understanding of the nature of nursing knowledge, to explore different ways of addressing the situation, partly through the introduction of a variety of new roles.

This book is concerned with exploring some of the underlying problems which have been highlighted by empirical work, but is focused on approaches that are being tried in order to overcome the difficulties. Experiences of people working in innovative roles, such as that of the lecturer practitioner and the clinician/lecturer are examined. Contributors have offered very real accounts of the way in which they have developed roles and shifted organizational structures in order to find ways of bringing together different aspects of professional work through unification.

The book is divided into four sections, each one offering a different perspective. Part One sets the scene by examining some of the background factors which are driving the changes. Following an introduction raising key areas of relevance it offers a comprehensive review of work which has been undertaken over the past two decades to explore ways which are conducive for students to learn about practice. This section also includes one author's fascinating insight into the way in which expert nurses practice.

In Part Two three authors share their experiences of establishing lecturer practitioner roles in Oxfordshire Health Authority. They have concentrated on recounting the work which was undertaken to establish a new way of functioning which meets the needs of both nursing practice and nurse education. In so doing they tell a story of change and development.

Part Three is the Australian experience where, in one faculty, there is an expectation that all staff will retain contact with practice, not only in a teaching but also in a learning capacity. If the essence of nursing work is to provide expert clinical care through practice then viable ways have to be found to maintain links between these two areas, and the authors of this section offer both the reasoning behind the changes and their experiences of reordering the responsibilities within their work.

Finally, Part Four of the book looks at some alternative approaches to integration. The way in which Nursing Development Units can contribute to integration is examined, as well as the value of job sharing. In the last chapter an attempt has been made to synthesize the key issues from the experiences outlined, and draw out the implications which may be of value for future developments.

The book has been prepared for those who have an interest in addressing the challenge of integration themselves. While the accounts mainly describe stories of success, no attempt has been made to hide the demands which many of the authors have faced in finding new ways of working. In sharing these experiences foundations can be set for future work.

Part One
Practice and Theory

1

Setting the scene

Barbara Vaughan

Introduction

There has been a growing acknowledgement over the past two decades that nursing practice is underpinned by a unique body of knowledge which guides expert clinicians (e.g. Watson, 1985; Perry and Jolley, 1991; Grey and Pratt, 1991). What is also becoming apparent is that much of this knowledge is not only unchartered but that it frequently goes unrecognized. Many reasons can be found to explain why such a situation has occurred: the division of labour which has arisen between nursing education, nursing management, nursing research and nursing practice; the lack of an adequate vocabulary to describe nursing; the inappropriateness of traditional research methods to explore nursing; and the complexity of caring itself are just a few. The challenge which we all face now is to find ways of moving forward in order to address some of these concerns.

The so called 'theory practice gap', which can be seen as a symptom of this situation, has been a subject of wide discussion (Lathlean, 1992). It is frequently suggested that there is a major discrepancy between what is said by those who teach nursing in a formal setting and those who practice nursing, which may give rise to conflict. It can, however, be argued that such a gap will always exist since there would be no progress if this was not the case. From this perspective it is a necessary prerequisite to change and development. Nevertheless it is unacceptable for formal education and practice to follow different paths. Not only will this lead to major dissonance for students but it can also act as a barrier to the development of nursing knowledge. Practice and education should be intertwined in such a way that theoretical propositions arise from practice itself, and that practice is informed by, and tests theory. Thus there is a need for mechanisms which allow for both inductive and deductive approaches to increase our understanding of nursing and inform the way in which we help students to gain expertise.

Moves are afoot on many sides to address these issues. Changes are occurring in educational programmes, organizational structures, national and local policy and, maybe most importantly in our understanding of the value and expertise in good practice (Royal College of Nursing, 1992; Audit Commission, 1991). The driving forces which have given rise to these reforms are complex in nature and stem from both internal and external sources. However it is important to gain an insight into them since this can serve to clarify the context in which the changes are occurring, and be of value in helping people find creative ways in which they can respond.

Changes in nurse education

The move, in the mid 1980s in Australia and more recently in the United Kingdom, to place student nurse programmes in institutes of higher education is maybe one of the most significant reforms of this century in nurse education. Firstly such a move gives formal acknowledgement to the complex nature of nursing knowledge which can be studied as an independent discipline. Secondly it has been accepted at last that the knowledge which all students gain during their preparatory training is worthy of recognition in academic terms. Thirdly it gives students of nursing access to people working in a wide range of other disciplines, thus broadening their horizons. Finally it opens up options for people working in other disciplines to learn more about nursing.

However, as is so often the case, such a positive move brings with it some hazards. Fears have been expressed that students will gain registration without adequate experience of practice; they will be lured into jobs distanced from patients or they will leave nursing for more prestigious work. Evidence of the career paths of nurse graduates to date (Bircumshaw and Chapman, 1988) contradicts these anxieties but they remain very real in some peoples minds.

What may be seen as more worrying is that shifting contracts of employment from health to educational organizations could lead to a widening of the gap between practitioners and educationalists unless active steps are taken to ensure that this is not the case. Sheer physical distance may make it more difficult for all those who teach nursing to retain a grasp of the reality of practice. Demands in higher education to reach research and publication goals may supersede the need to retain and refine clinical skills and while there is no recognition, in terms of staff–student ratios, of the need to teach practice these are very real concerns.

Similarly the move from a single discipline school of nursing to the multidiscipline educational setting brings with it a wealth of opportunity for access to knowledge from a wide range of other sources. There is, however, a parallel risk that nursing knowledge will get lost in the demand for curriculum time for physiology, psychology, sociology and all the other contributing subjects. As Street (1990) so aptly says;

> . . . in the professions least equipped with a secure foundation of systematic knowledge . . . yearning for the rigour of science based knowledge and power of science based techniques leads schools to import scholars from neighbouring departments of social sciences.

This situation has been made even more difficult to handle by the lack of opportunity until recent times for nurses to study to degree or higher degree level in their own discipline. In the 1970s and early 1980s many were deprived of the option of gaining advanced qualifications by studying nursing itself as the number of courses was so limited. In consequence the responsibility for teaching students to diploma or degree level often falls on the shoulders of people who have not had the experience themselves. Furthermore, despite the introduction of a new grading structure in the mid 1980s, the criteria for career advancement have remained largely managerial, forcing practitioners to move to roles based in management or education in order to advance their careers. Thus the opportunity to challenge, test and refine theory for themselves has frequently been lost.

In such a situation it becomes even more critical that ways are found to ensure that the practice of nursing is taught by those who are experts in their own field, that is skilled practitioners. Even with an acknowledgement that there will always be a gap between theory and reality the most complex thing we ask people to do is make sense of what they have learned through both experience and study. There is a critical difference between *applying* theory, which could be equated with the novice practitioner (Benner, 1984) and *using* theory to inform decision making in a creative way as a competent or expert practitioner (Benner, 1984). If we want to help students to grow beyond the level of novice then we must ensure that expert practitioners have some say in the development of their educational programmes.

Policy changes

All these advances are taking place against a rapidly moving scene where health policy is also changing. For many years we have lived in a society in which health services have been equated with the diagnosis and treatment of disease which, it can be argued, has created a dependency on health care professionals. Gradually a shift is occurring to redress this situation and the expectation that responsibility for health lies unchallenged with the medical profession alone is shifting.

Within a market driven environment health workers are being asked to account for their practice with identifiable targets in, for example, the *Patient's Charter* (Department of Health, 1991). Despite some concerns about the efficacy of offering a public service which is driven by market forces, the notion of public accountability has to be lauded. This principle should surely apply to all who offer such a service, implying that they have to be able to say what they do, why they do it and what the outcome of their actions is. For nurses this is a major challenge since, as an occupation, the degree of formal enquiry which has been undertaken is still limited. In an age when so much emphasis is being placed on the efficiency and effectiveness of services it is critical that ways are found of exploring and defining the interrelationship between nursing actions and patient outcomes. We do, however, have logical argument on our side and some evidence that experienced, qualified practitioners do improve the quality of care which patients receive (University of York, 1992).

Changes in emphasis towards primary health similarly open up opportunities to expand and evaluate the nursing contribution.

A further exciting policy initiative is the advent of health gain targets, aimed at reducing the incidence of disease, rather than curing those who are already afflicted, in 'Health for All' (Department of Health, 1992). With the skills that nurses already have in patient teaching, facilitating self-care and empowerment, rehabilitation and concern for individuals' right to choice, we are well placed to offer services in response to many of these goals. Indeed they reflect some of the basic humanistic values which underpin nursing.

The opportunities that these changes offer are great, but they carry with them a responsibility to be articulate about the way in which nursing practice impacts on patient outcomes. Saying objectively just what it is that nurses do which is so effective in empowering patients and helping them to heal is not easy, since we still have a limited vocabulary to describe some nursing interventions. Maybe one of the reasons why such a situation has occurred is that again there has been a separation between those who practise nursing and those who research. Furthermore many nursing practices do not lend themselves well to the traditional scientific research methods which have dominated enquiry for so long, and require new and innovative ways of evaluating both the effectiveness and the efficiency of the services.

There is, however, a growing body of evidence that experienced, qualified nurses have a direct impact on the quality of care which patients receive (e.g. Pearson *et al.*, 1992; University of York, 1992; Audit Commission, 1991). Nevertheless there is a vast amount of work to be undertaken in exploring the interrelationship between nursing actions and patient outcomes.

The combination of all these changes means that there is an increasing urgency for ways to be found which make public the impact of expert nursing. Not only should we be responding to national policy initiatives but also contributing to future directions in the provision of health care. There is an urgent need for those who are skilled in practice to proactively voice their opinions and ideas in order to inform both local and national policy. Many options are open to us, such as an increase in critical evaluation, placing people with clinical credibility on policy boards, learning to 'market' nursing and a greater degree of assertiveness, all of which potentially empower nurses to contribute more effectively.

Roles

The development of advanced clinical roles, such as that of the lecturer practitioner, is one specific way of helping skilled nurses to stay in close contact with clinical care while advancing their career and gaining the skills to contribute to policy. In this instance the responsibility for practice and education are predominant but research and management components are also evident. Indeed these four key elements, of practice, research, education and management can be combined in a variety of different ways to offer career paths which highlight the major interests of the incumbent while retaining a hold on all aspects of nursing work. Thus there is the researcher practitioner, the manager practitioner, the clinical nurse specialist and the nurse practitioner. All these roles are ways of unifying responsibility for different aspects of work and enhancing the integration of theory and practice.

Nursing, Midwifery and Health Visiting Development Units, supported by the government, are another way in which senior nurses can find a career path which brings together the various aspects of nursing work (Pearson, 1983; Vaughan, 1992). In this instance the units have a clearly identified *clinical* leader and a specific remit not only to seek excellence in practice but also to explore new ways of doing things: to evaluate their work; to act as a teaching and consultancy resource; to disseminate their findings and to have an input into policy making in their host organization. The skills required for such leadership are wide but there is increasing evidence of the efficacy of such a model for development (Pearson *et al.*, 1992).

There is no single right way in which Nursing Development Units (NDUs) develop but team involvement and ownership is critical (see Chapter 10). Thus there is opportunity for development not just of the clinical leader but of all the staff involved. Many team members take on responsibility for specific aspects of the development, generating ways of unifying different aspects of nursing work at an early stage in their career development.

Another role which impacts on unification is that of the primary nurse (Manthey, 1990). With more traditional ways of allocating work all managerial responsibility for the smooth running of clinical care was vested in the senior practitioner. With the responsibility for managing a case load, primary nurses have the opportunity of developing their managerial and leadership skills, as well as their clinical skills, at an earlier stage in their careers. An outcome of this move is that some of the work which was traditionally vested in the sister/charge nurse or clinical leader is delegated to primary nurses or team leaders, which in turn releases opportunities for changes in other nursing roles. It can be suggested that without a change of this nature many of the new roles described here would not be feasible. Role overload is already a serious issue which must be addressed and careful management is needed to restructure the order of things rather than just add on new aspects of work to a traditional role (Vaughan, 1990).

Developments in nursing knowledge

While there was a huge emphasis in the 1950s on the development of technical knowledge in health care the 1980s have brought with them a slow recognition of the importance of more humanistic needs (Bevis, 1978). Conceptual models have been described by many in an effort to bring to light frameworks which guide practice but there is still an urgent need to explore their efficacy and refine them in the light of experience. These changing ideologies that influence the direction in which both services and practice evolve bring with them an opportunity for nurses to expand and develop their understanding of the contribution they make to health care provision. While some will still argue that nursing knowledge is drawn from an amalgamation of 'borrowed' knowledge from other sources, this suggestion is widely disputed and there is a growing insight into the complex nature of the knowledge and skills which underpin practice (Grey and Pratt, 1991).

Research studies from the interpretative school are helping us to gain a better insight into effective nursing practices (e.g. Benner, 1984; MacLeod, 1990; Cahill, 1993) and laying foundations for further empirical work to assess the clinical management of such concepts as motivation, loss, caring and presencing (i.e. being with). However, it has to be acknowledged that these potential nursing diagnoses are difficult to grasp, especially by those who have no experience of them. Indeed, it can be suggested that one reason why people have chosen to move away from clinical work is to distance themselves from such issues which they find hard to address (cf. Kramer, 1974). Even though work in this area is old and valiant attempts have been made by many to ensure that they do build bridges between education and practice the difficulties remain very real.

Use of techniques such as *reflection in action* (Schön, 1987) and clinical supervision (Butterworth and Faugier, 1992) are helping to unravel the way in which nurses make clinical decisions and gain insight, not only into the knowledge they draw on but also the deficits in their understanding. However in order to facilitate such processes effectively it can be argued that expertise in practice and theory must be brought together. Certainly curricula need to be driven, research questions informed, and managerial structures developed, through the exploration of practice itself.

New nursing

'New nursing' has become a popular phrase in the 1990s (Salvage, 1988; Beardshaw and Robinson, 1990) yet much of what is talked about is a return to very traditional values. Caring itself is as old as time and certainly pre-empts the impact that science has had on health care. What is new is the growing insight which we are gaining of the primacy of practice, evidence of the development of new roles, the increase in interpretative and emancipatory research, the recognition of a discipline of nursing through validation of undergraduate to doctoral degrees and acknowledgement in national policy of the part which nurses have to play in the delivery of health care.

If these gains are to be sustained and advanced then ways must be found of ensuring that what is taught relates to practice, what is researched is founded on reality and that opportunities for developing and evaluating new and innovative ways of nursing are grasped. In the following chapters some approaches by which this challenge has been addressed are explored. In some ways the contributors are pioneers, moving into previously unknown territory. In other ways they are finding a means of bringing back to nursing much that was valued in the past but in a context which deals with a new pace and order of things.

References

Audit Commission (1991) *The Virtue of Patients: Making the Best Use of Ward Nursing Resources.* HMSO, London

Beardshaw, V. and Robinson, R. (1990) *New for Old – Prospects for Nursing in the 1990s.* King's Fund Research Report No. 8, King Edward's Hospital Fund for London

Benner, P. (1984) *From Novice to Expert: Excellence and Power in Clinical Nursing Practice.* Addison-Wesley, California

Bevis, E. (1978) *Curriculum Building in Nursing.* C. V. Mosby, St Louis

Bircumshaw, D. and Chapman, C. (1988) A follow up of the graduates of the Cardiff Bachelor of Nursing course. *Journal of Advanced Nursing,* **13** (2), 273–279

Butterworth, A. and Faugier, J. (1992) *Clinical Supervision and Mentorship in Nursing.* Chapman and Hall, London

Cahill, M. (1993) *Effective Nursing – An Exploration by Experienced Nurses.* Ashdale Press, Oxford

Department of Health (1991) *Patient's Charter.* Department of Health, London

Department of Health (1992) *Health of the Nation: A Strategy for Health in England.* HMSO, London

Grey, G. and Pratt, R. (1991) *Towards a Discipline of Nursing.* Churchill Livingstone, Edinburgh

Kramer, M. (1974) *Reality Shock: Why Nurses Leave Nursing.* C. V. Mosby, St Louis

Lathlean, J. (1992) The contribution of lecturer practitioners to theory and practice in nursing. *Journal of Clinical Nursing,* **1**, 237–242

MacLeod, M. (1990) Experience in Everyday Nursing Practice. A Study of 'Experienced' Ward Sisters. Unpublished PhD Thesis, University of Edinburgh

Pearson, A. (1983) *The Clinical Nursing Unit.* Butterworth-Heinemann, Oxford

Pearson, A., Punton, S. and Durant, E. (1992) *Nursing Beds – An Evaluation of The Effects of Therapeutic Nursing.* Scutari Press, London

Perry, A. and Jolley, M. (1991) *Nursing: A Knowledge Base for Practice*. Edward Arnold, London

Royal College of Nursing (1992) *The Value of Nursing*. RCN, London

Salvage, J. (1988) Partners in Care? An Exploration of the Theory and Practice of the New Nursing in the UK. MSc Thesis, Bedford and Royal Holloway College, University of London

Schön, D. A. (1987) *Educating the Reflective Practitioner*. Jossey-Bass, Oxford

Street, A. (1990) *Nursing Practice – High, Hard Ground, Messy Swamps and Pathways in Between*. Deakin University Press, Victoria

University of York Centre for Health Economics (1992) *Skill Mix and the Effectiveness of Nursing Care*. University of York Centre for Health Economics, York

Vaughan, B. (1990) Knowing that and knowing how: the role of the lecturer practitioner. In *Models for Nursing 2*. (eds J. Salvage and B. Kershaw). Scutari Press, London

Vaughan, B. (1992) The pursuit of excellence. *Nursing Times*, **88 (31)**, 26–28

Watson, J. (1985) *Nursing: The Philosophy and Science of Caring*. Colorado Associated University Press, Colorado

2

*Historical and empirical approaches**

Judith Lathlean

Introduction

Historically, issues about practice and theory in nursing have in the main been the preoccupations of nurse educators rather than of practitioners. Nevertheless, these concerns have always been pertinent to practitioners and this focus is reflected in some empirical work.

A glance at the literature shows that consideration of practice and theory has been pervasive. The notions are implicit if not explicit in the descriptions of nursing education from the time of Florence Nightingale through to contemporary writings on the subject. They are also embodied in the findings of much research, as well as being the focus of government reports, and the deliberations and recommendations of numerous committees considering the state and future direction of nurse education. Within the literature it is possible to determine three distinct but complementary approaches, especially, though not exclusively, in relation to educational aspects. First, practice–theory issues are expressed in terms of a problem, the nature of the problem is discussed and possible solutions are offered, but within the existing system. Second, proposals are made which are aimed at changing the whole system of nurse education and third, traditional roles are critiqued and new ones are suggested or even implemented (Lathlean, 1992). Finally, issues to do with theory

---

* This chapter represents an extension and modification of a review of 'theory practice' literature first published by Lathlean (1992).

and practice are germane within debates about the nature of nursing practice, knowledge and expertise, and can be viewed as axiomatic to current thinking about how professionals learn to become practitioners. Thus the chapter concludes with reference to some of the apposite literature in this respect.

Defining the problem

Empirical studies of nursing practice in the 1970s often concluded that there was a disparity between theory and observed practice (e.g. Hunt's (1974) study of the surgical dressing procedure, and Jones' (1975) research on nasogastric feeds), yet despite this highlighting of a disjunction, later studies showed similar patterns.

Most of the research, however, was from an education perspective. Some investigations focused on the relationship and ideological differences between school and service. For example, Bendall (1975), in a study of a sample of nurse training schools in England, concluded that there was a persistent dichotomy between what happened in the wards and what was prescribed in the syllabus, taught in the schools and questioned in the final examination. Dodd (1973) also suggested that the school was where students learnt to pass examinations and wards were where they learnt to nurse. She further observed that nurse teachers' values differed from the values of service nurses. This was also the finding of Pepper (1977) in a study focusing on professionalism, training and work.

Similarly, the theme of conflicting values emerged in research by Gott (1982). She studied three hospitals, concentrating on the relationship between nursing as taught in the school and as practiced in the ward, and concluded that 'in addition to failing to prepare student nurses for the skills expected of them, the ward teachers also failed to prepare them for the ideological conflict'. She identified two prevailing ideologies – professional and bureaucratic – and argued that the school subscribed to, although did not practise, the former, and the ward subscribed to the latter.

Melia (1987) also addressed these issues, and the tensions created in nursing between service needs and education. Based on student nurses' accounts of their experiences in training, she described nursing as an occupation with two fundamentally different views of its role, with education providing student nurses with an idealized, theoretical view of nursing, and the ward experiences emphasizing nursing as being about 'getting the work done'.

The integration of practice and theory

Other research concluded that practice and theory needed to be integrated more closely; for example, in Canada, Wong (1979) found an inability on the part of students to transfer classroom learning to clinical practice and Abdel-Al (1975) identified that students were expected to make the relationship themselves between practice and theory, and that their theoretical instruction did not reflect the complexity and variability of practice.

Attempts have been made to achieve greater integration. For example, Alexander (1983) conducted an experiment in Scotland, the aim of which was 'the facilitation of integration of theory and practice', but which assumed that the perceived problems were 'more likely to be a function of the methods of teaching and learning, than of the formal organisation of the training programme'. This study found that students considered that their training lacked integration: when practice was not realistically depicted in classroom teaching; when theory was not followed by relevant practice on the ward; when ward staff appeared to be unaware of the stage at which the student was at in terms of their training and experience; and when there was evidence of conflicting values between school and ward.

These findings in part appear to confirm a problem that had been identified earlier, and one that it was hoped would be ameliorated by the introduction of the modular system of training. For example, Bendall (1971) addressed the temporal relationship between theory and practice and concluded that the optimal solution was one where theory immediately preceded or followed practice, but there was little evidence of this occurring at the time of her study.

Alexander's (1983) experiment was deemed successful, and the ward-based supervised practice and the use of more experimental forms of learning were clearly considered to be beneficial by the students. Nevertheless, the approach used for the experiment perpetuated the situation whereby those with the prime responsibility for facilitating the students' learning about the practice of nursing – the tutors and clinical teachers – had no authority over the nature and standards of that practice.

In a later study, with remarkably similar aims and certain common features, McCaugherty (1991), using an action research methodology, developed and evaluated an experimental teaching model to promote integration of theory and practice by first-year students. However, despite the merits of this study the extent to which its success was dependent upon researcher intervention may well limit its wider generalizability, and again, it entailed a teacher entering a clinical area as a visitor.

The ward sister and clinical learning

In pursuit of a rather different tack, many researchers have concentrated on trying to understand what happens in ward and clinical situations in terms of clinical education. The main focus has been the role of the ward sister as a teacher, and the suitability of wards as areas for learning the practice of nursing.

The recognition that ward sisters should have a teaching role in relation to students is not new. Certainly it was recognized at the time of Florence Nightingale; in a memorandum drawn up in 1879 it was stated that – as part of her job – the sister 'trains the probationer nurses in their ward work both by direct instruction and by working with them' (Cope, 1955). Indeed, the importance attached to the educative function, the ways in which teaching is undertaken and learning occurs, the problems that are encountered and the beneficiaries of the teaching have been the focus of much attention in recent years – and the subject of considerable research.

The consensus of opinion from studies in the 1950s, 60s and early 70s was that sisters (and sometimes other trained ward staff) spent very little time with students. For example, in 1953, Goddard found that teaching had a low priority with trained staff, that sisters spent between 5 and 10% of their day in direct contact with students (half of which was for reports and instructions) and that formal teaching comprised only about 1% of the total time

(Nuffield Provincial Hospitals' Trust 1953). Revans (1964) found a similar situation, with sisters failing to teach and being perceived by learners as unapproachable and uncommunicative. This was reinforced by Lelean (1973) who, in a study of communication in three hospitals, showed that 60% of the ward sisters' communication was with staff nurses and only 3% with first-year student nurses. In a study concentrating initially on the educational role of the ward sister, Lamond (1974) discovered from students and qualified nurses that there was little consistency as to a single nurse rank being the ideal teacher, and that the sister was chosen in only little more than a third of the responses indicating the respondents choice of the best teacher in the ward situation.

These findings were supported by government reports in the 1960s. For example, a small scale study conducted by the Ministry of Health (1968) found that sisters spent less than 4% of their time in teaching and the Scottish Home and Health Department (1969) estimated that teaching averaged fifteen minutes a day. But it was often not the case that sisters were disinterested in teaching. Catnach and Houghton (1961) and MacGuire (1969) found there to be a discrepancy between the ideal teaching role expressed by sisters and the low priority accorded to ward teaching in reality, and Long (1976) showed that most of the sisters in her sample thought that they were in a good position to assess their learners and saw this, along with teaching, as part of their job, whilst the researcher doubted whether this was realistic. Furthermore, in a complex longitudinal study by Jacka and Lewin (1987), sisters, when questioned, tended to overestimate the amount of teaching and supervision that they – and their trained staff – provided.

Many reasons have been cited for this situation: the pressures of the ward work which made it difficult for sisters to devote adequate time to teaching and assessing (Exton-Smith, 1972), the inexperience of many sisters resulting in a tendency for them to lack confidence in their teaching ability (Bendall, 1971), and the general lack of preparation for this aspect of their role (Farnish, 1983).

However, some investigators have questioned the viability of the sister's teaching and assessment role; for example, Lelean (1973) suggested the sister's teaching role be reviewed and either her work be reorganized so that she has time to teach the student nurses or else it be accepted that teaching of students was done by others. The notion of 'formal' teaching has been challenged, and it has been suggested that ward staff and students learn as much if not more from sisters in other ways such as role modelling (e.g. Pembrey, 1980).

Another major aspect of empirical work in relation to clinical areas has been that which considers wards as learning environments. Much of the reasearch has recognized the ward sister as the key person in the creation of a good environment for learning on the ward, in particular Fretwell (1978) and Orton (1981). Orton (1983) suggested the existence of a measurable ward learning climate. She identified two entirely different types of ward which she labelled 'high student orientation' and 'low student orientation'. In the former, the characteristic features were the combination of teamwork, consultation and the sister's awareness of her subordinates' physical and emotional needs. Typically, the sister had a teaching programme, devoting a lot of time to students and using ward reports as valuable learning sessions. The converse prevailed in wards identified as low student orientation wards. Students were seen as pairs of hands rather than as learners, teaching was given low priority and potential learning opportunities were wasted. In pursuit of a somewhat different, though connected aspect, Ogier (1980) also investigated the role of the sister and concluded that sisters perceived as having a leadership style which is approachable were more favoured by students. She recommended that sisters be better prepared in interpersonal skills prior to taking charge of a ward.

The implications of such research on ward sisters is not so much one of a gap between theory and practice, but rather the ineffectiveness of clinical learning because the ward sister was not devoting sufficient time to teaching students. As a result of some of these studies, 'solutions' were posed to rectify the problem, an important one being the better preparation of sisters for their roles including the teaching aspects (e.g. see Lathlean and Farnish, 1984).

Wards as learning areas

Given the concern about the potential of wards as places in which to learn about nursing, it is perhaps surprising that few studies have directly considered the problem of how to develop criteria to assess wards as learning areas. In a major project which did address this problem, Jacka and Lewin (1987) reviewed the limited research in this area. They cited the study of Martin (1976) which discusses the conflict between educational and service needs, offering general guidelines about converting the learner's daily work into 'clinical learning experiences'. These include careful selection of the learning area, opportunity in the ward for observation and adequate practice, and helpful communication and feedback. The work of Shröck (1973), undertaken on a much larger scale, is also germane. Shröck studied a large hospital group specializing in mental illness and mental handicap and aimed to develop a method of continuous evaluation of clinical areas suitable for training. Her research resulted in the development of a 'ward profile' designed to give reliable information about a ward's learning opportunities and she concluded, perhaps unsurprisingly, that wards with a common designation (as to their type) do not all have similar characteristics.

Shröck's study was supported by the work of Roper (1976). She investigated the clinical conditions of patients in thirty-one wards and concluded that the medical label given by the ward was misleading. So, for example, she found that 39% of patients in a general hospital had more than one medical label, and that ward labels such as 'paediatric' and 'geriatric' were confusing, since there were children and elderly patients in most wards of the hospital. Roper pointed out the implications for nurse education, whereby a student nursing in one such ward is likely to encounter a wider range of nursing situations than superficially apparent.

In a study in Northern Ireland, Reid (1985) investigated how to determine the suitability of a clinical area for nurse training, and how to estimate what number of learners could be effectively taught there. Despite these studies, there has been a relative paucity of research into student clinical learning and few guidelines available to assist those concerned with improving the educational quality of clinical allocation. This deficiency was the stimulus for the project, conducted over a period of several years, by Jacka and Lewin (1987). In a methodologically novel study, they 'investigated three training schemes and the experiences of those within them, the ultimate aim being to show a way to improvement of existing methods and arrangements whereby students are enabled to acquire knowledge and skill necessary for competence in nursing practice within a hospital'. Through their research they developed a method for calibrating the clinical experience of student nurses and the relationship between 'instruction' and practice. They concluded that they see 'the construction of methods for monitoring opportunity and experience as [their] central contribution'.

Changing the system

Whilst much of the foregoing research offers 'solutions' to the bridging of the theory practice gap, or the better integration of theory and practice in some way, the emphasis is on changing often a small part of the system rather than the whole. Thus even where change has been attempted this is rarely the answer to quite fundamental and long-standing problems. In the wake of such empirical and other evidence, it has been argued that the only way to overcome the problems is by radical innovation whereby the entire system is reviewed and developed.

Martin (1989), in considering the system of nurse education over the past century, identifies two major factors that have dominated the way in which nurses have been educated – the apprenticeship system and its implications for the staffing of hospitals and the 'interplay that developed and still exists between the government, the nursing statutory bodies and the professional oraganizations about policies for nurses education'. Perhaps because of this dominance change in the whole approach to nurse education has been slow.

Two documents – the Platt Report (Royal College of Nursing, 1964) and the Briggs Report (Department of Health and Social Security, 1972) – addressed the issue of the gap between theory and practice and the need to provide better clinical learning for students. Neither of these reports was implemented at the time, though the recommendations of the Brigg's Committee especially have been influential in informing the current reform in nurse education in the United Kingdom – Project 2000 (United Kingdom Central Council, 1986). In addition, the Royal College of Nursing (RCN) Commission, under the chairmanship of Dr Harry Judge, in its report highlighted the 'central error of treating learners as an integral part of the workforce' and the 'uneasy relationship between tutors on the one hand and ward staff on the other' (Royal College of Nursing, 1985). It acknowledged certain 'solutions', as discussed later, but suggested that clinical teachers had been 'unevenly introduced as antidotes or mediators and joint appointments [were] merely mooted'. Rather than 'an elaboration of detail', it argued for the assertion of structural principles, by far the most important being 'an overdue re-definition of the relationship between education, clinical experience and service'. It further suggested that this would be best achieved by 'placing nurse education within the flexible framework of higher education itself' (Royal College of Nursing, 1985).

As Lathlean (1989) pointed out, in an empirical study of the way in which policy decisions were made in relation to the current changes in nurse education (United Kingdam Central Council, 1986), 'it is difficult to know how much influence the recommendations of the [RCN] Commission had on the outcome of educational reform, but some . . . felt it acted as an important catalyst'. Project 2000 itself (United Kingdom Central Council, 1986) recognized a theory practice problem, and talked about the common core foundation programme as being a 'theory and practice' programme and not one solely concerned with theory, with placements being 'planned systematically so that theory can be applied critically by students in different practice settings'. However, it has been argued that, 'without further changes to the system, such statements do little in themselves to overcome the disparity between theory and practice' (Lathlean, 1992).

The development and implementation of new roles

Alongside the major reform of the system there have been many attempts to overcome the problems by the introduction of new roles. The main ones have been clinical teachers, joint appointments and more recently, lecturer practitioners. (Other variants are described in this book, but there has been little or no empirical evidence as to their implementation and effectiveness).

The clinical teacher

In the late 1950s the specialized role of clinical instructor – later called the clinical teacher – was introduced to help students integrate theory and practice and to supervise their clinical practice. Whilst many anecdotal descriptions have been published, particularly generated by clinical teachers themselves, little research existed until it became evident that there were problems with the role. In a survey by Kirkwood (1979), three quarters of the clinical teachers in the sample were found to be unhappy with the role, with almost a quarter planning to train as tutors and 14% to go into administration. Kirkwood suggested that their dissatisfaction was primarily due to feelings of low status and to a perception that they had no clearly differentiated role.

This study supported many of the findings of an earlier large-scale survey of registered teachers of nursing (General Nursing Council, 1975), which indicated the three most common concerns amongst clinical teachers as: inadequate recognition of the clinical teacher's job; the conflict between education and service; and the inadequate definition of responsibility. Similarly, Martin (1989), whilst examining in the mid 1970s 'the role and status of clinical teachers within the context of policies for nurse education', and Robertson (1987), who conducted a survey of one school of nursing and its associated hospitals in the early 1980s, concluded that problems stemmed from the perceptions of others about clinical teaching, and the way in which it was organized and implemented. Wright (1981), in a descriptive survey using questionnaires and interviews in five schools of nursing, also found there to be considerable dissatisfaction with the role, both amongst clinical teachers and members of their role set. Wright highlighted the problem of role strain and conflict related to their dual role as teachers and nurses, and concluded that 'in general they are accepted by neither the school as fully developed teachers nor the ward as fully responsible nurses'.

Whilst it is argued that the need for clinical teaching remains, the United Kingdom Central Council for Nurses, Midwives and Health Visitors has decreed that there should be a single grade of teacher rather than the two (United Kingdom Central Council, 1986), and it ceased to recognize new qualifications for clinical teachers after September 1987.

Joint appointments

Another 'organizational solution' – suggested in the Briggs Report (Department of Health and Social Security, 1972) and in the Royal Commission on the National Health Service (1979, para 13.43) as a method of bridging the gap between education and service – is that of joint appointments. They can take on a variety of forms, but one occupant of such a role suggests that there are four themes in the functioning of a joint appointee:

1 He or she works as a teacher in both the school and the ward, demonstrating nursing, management and research skills and acting as a specialist resource.
2 He or she brings together the roles of trained teacher and practising trained nurse in charge of care.
3 He or she acts as manager of the ward and its staff. This includes the organizing of work, supervising resources, counselling, guiding and coordinating the activities of staff.
4 He or she will develop research into nursing (Wright, 1983).

Clearly jobs with such features are aimed at the closer integration of nursing theory and practice.

A report of a peer group of nurses working in combined teaching and clinical roles, and researchers with an interest in the role (King's Fund, 1984), included: an appraisal of joint appointments, giving examples such as a joint university/NHS appointment (Ashworth and Castledine, 1980); a description of what joint appointees do; views of the posts from different perspectives such as those of students and managers, and the effects of joint appointments on patients, clients and relatives. However, although the King's Fund report is illuminative of several of the relevant issues – and it concluded that many such post holders felt that they had achieved a considerable amount for the education of learner nurses – it is primarily descriptive rather than analytic.

References about joint appointments are prolific – a computer-based search of the literature produced well over fifty – but there has been little systematic evaluation of the concept or research in the area. One exception to this is a study by Balogh and Bond (1984), whereby two appointees were evaluated, each working half the time as ward sister and the other half as clinical teacher and nurse tutor respectively. Although there were many positive aspects to this arrangement, it was found that 'the joint appointment itself became an object of anxiety over the duration of the project, and the partners became separately identified in the minds of the staff within the school and the service area. In addition the organization of the appointment did not provide for any circumstances under which the split could be unified'. The researchers pointed out that their study confirms the observations of other joint appointees (Ashworth and Castledine, 1980; Walden *et al.*, 1982).

Whilst studies of the clinical teacher concentrate on the role of a clinically based teacher whose rationale for existence is clinical teaching, and studies of joint appointments focus on appointees who have joint education and service responsibilities, a third variation has been highlighted by Hawker and Kevern (1987). They have reported on an exploratory 'qualitative' study of four nurse teachers who transferred their base from the school to the ward area, and they argue that despite the practical and personal difficulties encountered, the role of the ward based teacher can be intrinsically rewarding and its scope far reaching. They suggested – using role theory – that the ward-based teacher uses the sources of role fulfilment in a role set as reinforcers to reduce the strains created by the conflicting demands of the teacher's commitment to the school and the ward.

Lecturer practitioners

The idea of lecturer practitioners has arisen both to ameliorate the problems experienced with other approaches and as an alternative which, ideally, is designed to be an integral part of a new system of managing nursing practice and facilitating nurse education. It stemmed from 'concern about the difficulties experienced by both practitioners and educators in finding a match between what was being done in practice and what was being taught in theory, as well as a fundamental belief in the value of practice as the origin of much nursing theory' (Vaughan, 1990). Although lecturer practitioner jobs exist in a number of health authorities and colleges of nursing and midwifery, there appears to be as yet only one health authority – Oxfordshire – where lecturer practitioners in large numbers (currently more than seventy) are an integral part of both the nursing service structure and the educational institution (Champion, 1992). Though the experiences of three of these lecturer practitioners are described in this book, little empirical work exists on these roles, apart from the action research study that one of them made of her own role in order to be more analytical about her practice and the effect of her actions (FitzGerald, 1989). Another exception is a major four-year research study that is being undertaken by Judith Lathlean of the implementation and development of the roles. This research comprises a longitudinal in-depth ethnographic case study of a small number of lecturer practitioners, complemented by an analysis of the perspectives of those working most closely with them, and a survey of the views of all of the lecturer practitioners across the organization

Whilst the whole project has still to be completed, some preliminary findings about the lecturer practitioner's role in relation to issues of theory and practice are reported in Lathlean (1992). It seems from this study that lecturer practitioners 'do not see their task as bridging a theory–practice gap [as such]. Rather, their actions stem from their joint clinical and education responsibilities, and the integral relationship between them'. They all have 'a major part to play in the development of the clinical areas in which they operate, and especially through their relationships with the ward staff'. And, in this process, they are 'conscious . . . of using their knowledge and skills to enhance practice for the intrinsic benefits this brings for the care of the patients, in order to assist the ward staff to be better practitioners and to provide good examples of nursing for students to learn from'. As they do so, 'they frequently draw on theoretical work, as well as theorising about what they are doing' (Lathlean, 1992).

In addition, there are a number of other ways in which lecturer practitioners facilitate the integration of theory and practice, for example, through their involvement with the curriculum development for the students' practice modules, the organization of students' learning in clinical placements, the encouragement of reflection on practice by clinicians acting as mentors and by students, and by the part they play in the assessment of students through discussion of their learning contracts. (These issues are elaborated upon in later chapters.)

Alternative perspectives

So far the review has concentrated on the substantial literature indicating ways in which practice–theory issues have been identified, and solutions that have been proposed by means of new roles or by the reform of the system. There are, however, at least two other areas of work where issues of theory and practice are pertinent – the development and understanding of the nature of nursing practice, and the related attempts to analyse how nurses and other professionals learn to practice. Both will only be touched upon briefly here, though many of the concepts are evident throughout this book.

The nature of nursing practice has been the subject of considerable debate, much of which is to do with trying to ascertain what is nursing knowledge and how nurses become knowledgeable about practice. This implies a move on, or at least away from the idea of a gap between 'theory' or the knowledge base of nursing and the practice of nursing, to an attempt to understand more precisely the differences between practical and theoretical knowledge.

Currently, a distinction is increasingly being made between 'knowing' and 'knowledge'. For example, Schultz and Meleis (1988) suggest that nursing practice is informed both by intuitive knowing and by systematically verified knowledge. Knowledge in nursing has been deemed by Carper (1978) to have four aspects – empirical, aesthetical, personal and ethical – and Cahill (1993) compares the empirical aspect with the systematically verified knowledge and the other three with intuitive knowing. Intuitive knowing is also likened to Polyani's (1962) notion of 'tacit knowledge' or intellectual know-how. Others describe similar concepts of knowledge in practice; for example, Schön (1983) talks about 'knowing-in-action' for professionals and Benner (1984) makes reference to 'knowledge embedded in practice' in the context of nursing.

Amongst the wealth of theoretical literature related to nursing in this respect, three research studies emerge as innovative examples, or attempts to explore the issues further. Benner (1984) builds on the work by Dreyfus and Dreyfus (1986) on how airline pilots acquire and develop skill. Her aim within nursing was to 'examine the differences between practical and theoretical knowledge; provide examples of competencies from the study of nursing practice; describe aspects of practical knowledge; and outline strategies for preserving and extending that knowledge' (Benner, 1984). She distinguishes between the novice nurse, whose behaviour is dependent on specific knowledge and the demonstration of specific skills and the increasingly competent nurse, whose behaviour is the result of an amalgam of knowledge and skills, related to a context and decreasingly explicit in its practice–theory elements, and argues that nurses move through five identifiable stages in the process of acquiring expertise.

MacLeod (1990), clearly influenced by the work of Benner (1984), takes the ideas on further by examining the nature of everyday experience for nurses and how this contributes to the development of nursing expertise. Her aim in the research is both to understand the nature of learning to nurse and the development of expertise, and consequently to identify how such understandings can inform the better preparation of nurses. In doing so she calls for 'a reformulation of the traditional distinctions of theory and practice'. (The findings and implications of this study are more fully described in Chapter 3.) Most recently, Cahill (1993) has sought to offer a description of 'effective nursing', through the use of a hermeneutic phenomenological approach, from the perceptions of seven experienced clinical nurses working in psychiatric and general care settings. Importantly, it 'reveals the crucial place of clinical knowledge developed through practice in the expertise of nurses and suggests ways for nursing practice to become central to both initial and continuing education of nurses' (Cahill, 1993). And, as with MacLeod's work, it offers a reconceptualization of theory practice for nursing.

Sometimes the aim of such thinking and investigation has been most specifically to do with the education of professionals and the part played by experience. For example, Argyris and Schön (1974) argue that 'practice must be made central to professional education rather than peripheral to it'. Later work by Schön (1983), in respect of the education of a number of different professionals, led to an analysis of the epistemology of professional practice which opposes 'reflective' to the more common 'technocratic' model of practice. In other words, he makes a distinction between professional knowledge as the application of science and professional knowledge as derived from practice, with the latter having historically been of low status. But Schön challenges the appropriateness of this and says that in practice, as in everyday life, our knowing is embedded in our action, and 'reflection-in-action' involves becoming conscious of the tacit 'knowledge' incorporated in the routines of practice, and subjecting that 'knowledge' to critical examination as it is used to make sense of situations of uncertainty and uniqueness. Further, Schön (1987) argues that professional education should be centred on enhancing the practitioner's ability for 'reflection-in-action', that is learning by doing and developing the ability for continued learning and problem solving throughout the professional's career. Again this challenges traditional notions of theory and practice, and their place in the education and training of professionals.

Conclusion

It is evident from the literature that issues of theory and practice have been an important concern within nursing for decades. Traditionally they have often been viewed as distinct entities, with theory achieving a higher status than practice, and with a perennial problem being that of a gap between the two. Many have sought to bridge that gap by more or less radical solutions. However, some have attempted to challenge that conceptualization, especially by examining the fundamentals of nursing itself – the nature of knowledge for nursing practice, and the processes by which nurses learn how to practice and the development of expertise.

References

Abdel-Al, H. (1975) Relating Education to Practice Within a Nursing Context. Unpublished PhD Thesis, University of Edinburgh

Alexander, M. F. (1983) *Learning to Nurse: Integrating Theory and Practice*. Churchill Livingstone, Edinburgh

Argyris, C. and Schön, D (1974) *Theory in Practice: Increasing Professional Effectiveness*. Jossey Bass, San Francisco

Ashworth, P. and Castledine, G. (1980) Joint service/education appointments in nursing. *Medical Teacher*, 2, 295–299

Balogh, R. and Bond, S. (1984) An analytical study of a joint clinical teaching/service appointment on a hospital ward. *International Journal of Nursing Studies*, 21 (2), 81–91

Bendall, E. (1971) The Learning Process in Student Nurses: Some Problems and Variables. Unpublished MA Thesis, University of London

Bendall, E. (1975 *So You Passed, Nurse*. Royal College of Nursing, London

Benner, P. (1984) *From Novice to Expert: Excellence and Power in Clinical Nursing Practice*. Addison-Wesley, California

Cahill, M. (1993) *Effective Nursing – An Exploration by Experienced Nurses*. Ashdale Press, Oxford

Carper, B. A. (1978) Fundamental patterns of knowing in nursing. *Advances in Nursing Science*, **1** (1), 13–23

Catnach, A. and Houghton, M. (1961) *Report of Pilot Investigation into Methods of Teaching in Nurse-Training Schools*. London-South West Metropolitan Area Nurse Training Committees

Champion, R. (1992) Professional collaboration: the lecturer practitioner role. In *Developing Professional Education* (eds H. Bines and D. Watson), The Society for Research into Higher Education and Open University Press, Buckingham

Cope, Z. (1955) *A Hundred Years of Nursing at St Mary's Hospital, Paddington*. Heinemann, London

Department of Health and Social Security (1972) *Report of the Committee on Nursing* (Chairman: Briggs). HMSO, London

Dodd, A. P. (1973) Towards an Understanding of Nursing. Unpublished PhD Thesis, University of London

Dreyfus, H. L. and Dreyfus, S. E. with Athanasiou, T. (1986) *Mind Over Machine: The Power of Human Intuition and Expertise in the Era of the Computer*. The Free Press, New York

Exton-Smith, J. (1972) Management of ward-based assessments. *Nursing Times*, **9**, 349–350

Farnish, S. (1983) *Ward Sister Preparation: a Survey in Three Districts*. NERU Report 2, Chelsea College, University of London

FitzGerald, M. (1989) Lecturer Practitioner: Action Researcher. Unpublished MN Thesis, Cardiff University

Fretwell, J. (1978) Socialisation of Nurses: Teaching and Learning in Hospital Wards. Unpublished PhD Thesis, University of Warwick

General Nursing Council for England and Wales (1975) *Teachers of Nursing*. GNC, London

Gott, M. (1982) Learning Nursing: A Study of the Effectiveness and Relevance of Teaching Provided During Student Nurse Introductory Course. Unpublished PhD Thesis, University of Hull

Hawker, R. and Kevern, J. (1987) *The Ward Based Teacher: An Exploratory Study*. Papers for a King's Fund Conference, King's Fund, London

Hunt, J. (1974) *The Teaching and Practice of Surgical Dressings in Three Hospitals*. Royal College of Nursing, London

Jacka, K. and Lewin, D. (1987) *The Clinical Learning of Student Nurses*. Nursing Education Research Unit, King's College, University of London

Jones, D. (1975) *Food for Thought*. Royal College of Nursing, London

King Edward's Hospital Fund for London (1984) *Joint Clinical-Teaching Appointments in Nursing*. King's Fund, London

Kirkwood, L. (1979) The clinical teacher. *Nursing Times*, 75 (12), 49–51 (Occasional Papers)

Lamond, N. (1974) *Becoming a Nurse: The Registered Nurses' View of the General Student Nurse Education*. Royal College of Nursing, London

Lathlean, J. and Farnish, S. (1984) *The Ward Sister Training Project*. Nursing Education Research Unit, Chelsea College, University of London

Lathlean, J. (1989) *Policy Making in Nurse Education*. Ashdale Press, Oxford

Lathlean, J. (1992) The contribution of lecturer practitioners to theory and practice in nursing. *Journal of Clinical Nursing*, 1, 237–242

Lean, S. (1973) *Ready for Report Nurse?* Royal College of Nursing, London

Long, P. (1976) Judging and reporting on student nurse clinical performance: some problems for the ward sister. *International Journal of Nursing Studies*, 13, 115–121

MacGuire, J. (1969) *Threshold to Nursing*. G. Bell and Sons, London

MacLeod, M. (1990) Experience in Everyday Nursing Practice. A Study of 'Experienced' Ward Sisters. Unpublished PhD Thesis, University of Edinburgh

Martin, J. L. (1976) Learning through experience. *Nursing Times*, 72 (14), 546–548

Martin, L. (1989) *Clinical Education in Perspective*. Royal College of Nursing, London

McCaugherty, D. (1991) The use of a teaching model to promote reflection and the experimental integration of theory and practice in first-year student nurses: an action research study. *Journal of Advanced Nursing*, 16, 534–543

Melia, K. (1987) *Learning and Working: The Occupational Socialization of Nurses*. Tavistock Publications, London

Ministry of Health (1968) *Nursing Work in General Hospital Wards*, HMSO, London

Nuffield Provincial Hospitals Trust (1953) *The Work of Nurses in Hospital Wards: Report of a Job Analysis*. (ed. Goddard, H. A.). Nuffield Provincial Hospitals Trust, London

Ogier, M. (1980) A Study of the Ward Sister's Leadership Style and Verbal Interaction with Nurse Learners. Unpublished PhD Thesis, University of London

Orton, H. (1981) Ward learning climate and student nurse response. *Nursing Times*, 77 (17), 65–68 (Occasional Paper)

Orton, H. (1983) Ward learning climate and student response. In *Research into Nurse Education* (ed. B. Davis). Croom Helm, Kent

Polyani, M. (1962) *Personal Knowledge – Towards a Post-Critical Philosophy*. Routledge and Kegan Paul, London

Pembrey, S. (1980) *The Ward Sister – Key to Nursing*. Royal College of Nursing, London

Pepper, R. J. (1977) Professionalism, Training and Work. Unpublished PhD Thesis, University of Kent

Reid, N. G. (1985) *Wards in Chancery? Nurse Training in the Clinical Area*. Royal College of Nursing, London

Revans, R. W. (1964) *Standards for Morale: Cause and Effect in Hospitals*. Oxford University Press, London

Robertson, C. M. (1987) *The Development and Practice of Clinical Teaching*. Royal College of Nursing, London

Roper, N. (1976) *Clinical Experience in Nurse Education*. Churchill Livingstone, Edinburgh

Royal College of Nursing (1964) *A Reform of Nursing Education: Report of a Special Committee on Nurse Education* (Chairman: Platt). Royal College of Nursing, London

Royal College of Nursing (1985) *The Education of Nurses: A New Dispensation. Commission on Nursing Education* (Chairman: Judge). Royal College of Nursing, London

Royal Commission on the National Health Service (1979) *Royal Commission on the National Health Service* (Merrison Report). HMSO (Cmnd 7615), London

Schön, D. (1983) *The Reflective Practitioner: How Professionals Think in Action*. Temple Smith, London

Schön, D. (1987) *Educating the Reflective Practitioner: Towards a New Design for Teaching and Learning in the Professions*. Jossey-Bass, San Francisco

Schröck, R. A. (1973) No rhyme of reason: a clinical area identification project. *International Journal of Nursing Studies*, **10**, 69–80

Schultz, P. R. and Meleis, A. F. (1988) Nursing epistemology: traditions, insights, questions. *Image: Journal of Nursing Scholarship*, **20** (4), 217–221

Scottish Home and Health Department (1969) *Nursing Workload as a Basis for Staffing*. (Scottish Health Service Studies 9). Scottish Home and Health Department

United Kingdom Central Council For Nursing Midwifery and Health Visiting (1986) *Project 2000: A New Preparation for Practice*. UKCC, London

Vaughan, B. (1990) Knowing that and knowing how: the role of the lecturer practitioner. In *Models for Nursing 2*. (eds J. Salvage and B. Kershaw). Scutari Press, London

Walden, E., Gallant, K. and Sander, R. (1982) Sharing the pain and the pleasure. *Nursing Times*, **78**, 833–837

Wong, J. (1979) The inability to transfer learning to clinical nursing practice: a learning problem and its remedial plan. *Journal of Advanced Nursing*, **4**(2), 161–168

Wright, S. G. (1981) The Role of the Clinical Teacher in General Nursing. Unpublished MSc Thesis, University of Manchester

Wright, S. G. (1983) Joint appointments 3: the best of both worlds. *Nursing Times*, **79**, 25–29

3

The everyday experience of nursing practice

Martha MacLeod

Introduction

Nursing practice is increasingly acknowledged to be a complex, multifaceted endeavour in which the competence of the nurse determines the quality of nursing care received by the patient or client. Although the need for knowledgeable, experienced nurses has been well established, there is less agreement on how to prepare nurses, both at entry and advanced levels. Perhaps this is not surprising, as the nature of learning to nurse and the development of nursing expertise is so imperfectly understood.

Learning has long been studied within educational contexts, but learning that is independent of efforts to educate has received scant attention, even within the adult learning literature (Thomas, 1986). Such 'natural' learning occurs in the midst of ongoing, everyday activities. It is common for us, working day-by-day, to experience a deepening of knowledge and an increase in our range of skills and abilities. Indeed, we may extend our knowledge and skill without any direct attention to the learning that we do. We take it for granted.

Such 'taken-for-granted' experience provides the basis for this chapter. The discussion arises from an interpretative study of the nature of everyday experience and its contribution to the development of nursing expertise (MacLeod, 1990). The nature of knowing, and its development in nurses' everyday experience of clinical nursing practice, is the focus.

Everyday experience provides a useful 'window' to knowing in nursing. Through an examination of everyday experience, formal knowledge can be gained about the substance of nursing practice, what Meleis (1987) calls 'the business of nursing'.

The substance of nursing lies in those caring practices which help people '. . . in the performance of those activities contributing to health, or its recovery (or to a peaceful death) that they would perform unaided if they had the necessary strength, will, or knowledge' (Henderson, 1966). Such caring practices are often difficult to talk about because of their complexity and the reliance on the context in which they take place for their meaning (Kitson, 1987). But as Benner (Benner, 1984; Benner and Wrubel, 1989) illustrates so richly, an examination of nurses' experiences reveals the knowledge and skills embedded in their practices.

Consideration of everyday experience also reveals knowledge about the development of clinical competence. Experience in clinical practice is considered to be essential to developing nursing knowledge and skills, as nursing is a practice-based profession (United Kingdom Central Council, 1987). McFarlane (1977) reminds us of our impressions of the wisdom of experienced ward sisters, and Benner (1984) argues convincingly that the development of expertise is not limited to, but is directly connected to experience. Thus, it would seem reasonable that an examination of ongoing, moment-by-moment experience would provide a glimpse of the way in which knowing in nursing practice develops.

Exploring everyday experience

In the study (MacLeod, 1990) which forms the basis for this chapter, the everyday experience in nursing practice of ten 'excellent, experienced' nurses in two Scottish hospitals was uncovered and explored. They were identified by the hospitals' Directors of Nursing Services, and met criteria adapted from Benner (1984) to identify expert nurses*. Since eight were ward sisters, and the other two were staff nurses who fulfilled part of a ward sister role, they are collectively referred to throughout as the

---

* ● Employed in nursing clinical practice for at least five years.
  ● Currently engaged in direct patient care in a surgical nursing setting.
  ● Identified by colleagues as highly skilled clinical practice nurses.
  ● Employed full-time in nursing.
  ● Registered general nurses.

'Sisters'. The ward sister is generally thought to be the 'repository of clinical expertise' (Lathlean, 1987) and locating experience and excellence in clinical practice at this position is not unusual in the National Health Service.

The Sisters were very experienced: they had been qualified between six and thirty-three years and had been in their current posts between two and a half and twelve years. They worked on general surgery, ear, nose and throat, gynaecology, orthopaedic trauma, thoracic surgery, urology and vascular surgery wards. Each was given a pseudonym which has been retained in this chapter.

The interpretative approach

The interpretative approach behind this research and discussion can be traced to the philosophical work of Heideggar (1962), who offers a radically different way of understanding human activity and experience. He suggests that peoples' actions and experiences are not a combination of objective properties and subjective beliefs, feelings and perceptions. He proposes instead, that human existence is better understood to be historical and intersubjective in nature. Our language and taken-for-granted actions show that we cannot be disconnected from our surroundings, from each other and from the influence of time. Studies which concentrate on subjective beliefs or objective properties fail to capture this complexity of human experience.

One of Heidegger's examples illustrates the everyday skilful coping in taken-for-granted experience. When we open a door, we are not aware of turning the doorknob, we are only aware of the doorknob when it sticks. When the doorknob sticks we attempt to unstick it, and it is only when that does not work that we may need to think about the specific properties of the doorknob itself. Heidegger argues that what needs study before the problem of knowing, is everyday being-in-the world, as 'much if not most characteristic human activity is not guided by conscious choices, and not accompanied by aware states of mind' (Magee, 1987). It would follow then, that much of everyday experience in nursing practice is overlooked and taken for granted because it is skilful coping in the midst of an ongoing situation. Unless a problem develops, or a doorknob sticks, we remain unaware of the skills and knowledge essential to this coping. Thus an approach following in the tradition of Heidegger, hermeneutic phenomenology, may be a more fruitful way of examining everyday, taken-for-granted nursing experience.

Many studies have sought to identify the objective properties of nursing practice or knowledge (e.g. Pembrey, 1980; Kitson, 1986; Seers, 1987). Other studies have focused on the subjective feelings, beliefs or perceptions of nurses about aspects of their practice (cf. Runciman, 1983). Studies of nursing experience (e.g. Field, 1981; Forrest, 1989) frequently maintain the distinction between subjective and objective data, as do studies of learning through experience (cf. Argyris and Schön, 1974; Jarvis, 1987; Griffin, 1987). Several sociological studies of nursing work and experience (cf. Strauss *et al.*, 1985; Melia, 1987; Smith, 1988) move quickly from an analysis of subjective experience to an explanation of the underlying social processes. While all such studies make important contributions to our understanding of nursing practice, experience and learning, they leave some important gaps.

Studies which use hermeneutic phenomenology (e.g. Gray-Snelgrove, 1982; Benner, 1984; Diekelmann, 1988) seem to be more successful at capturing the complex nature of learning, experience and nursing practice. For example Benner's (Benner, 1984; Benner and Wrubel, 1989) research reveals the ongoing context of practice of which tasks are but a part: the goals and meaning of practice; the knowledge and decision-making skills required to care for patients in an appropriate and timely manner; the interconnected nature of the individual and the social world. Through this interpretative approach the richness and complexity of nursing experience, practice and knowledge can be revealed.

Field work

The field work for this study took place over an eleven-month period, consisting of seven days of participant observation and three interviews with each Sister. In addition a group interview was also carried out.

Two principles were touchstones throughout the research. First, attention was focused on the *nurse-in-practice*, not on the nurse *removed from a context*, nor on the *context without the nurse*. Second, endeavours were made to *keep close* to experience, to continually ask while in the field and during interpretation, 'What does this mean about experience?'.

A hermeneutic interpretation

The interview transcripts and field notes were treated as text, or text analogues and a *hermeneutic interpretation* carried out (Gadamer, 1975; Ricoeur, 1979; Rabinow and Sullivan, 1979). Hermeneutics is an 'attempt to make clear, to make sense of an object of study' (Taylor, 1971). The meaning of an action or text (or text analogue) does not rest only in the writer, actor or speaker, nor in the interpreter alone, but is constituted in both. The interpretation sought was not just the Sisters' own interpretation. Instead, an attempt was made to bring to light what the Sisters already understood about their experience and practices, but in a new way, in a new interpretation, one *beyond* their own.

Insights into experience

In the course of the interviews, the Sisters described in some detail their experiences in nursing and of people they had nursed. As they were shadowed in practice, they would sometimes comment on what they were doing, either spontaneously or in response to a question. Perhaps what is most striking in their accounts is how elusive and fluid experience seems to be, and how much of their everyday practice is taken for granted and is therefore missing from the accounts.

The interviews gave insights into the Sisters' experiences of practice in the past, their comments on recent practice, and connections which they were able to make (or not able to make) between current and past practices. When observing practice, it can be assumed that experience is being drawn on. However, no one can determine what aspects of today's practice will join that ever-changing, amorphous body that they refer to as their 'experience'. Although there are some exceptions, it is difficult to say what portions of current practice appear to be drawing on past experience. The connection is not and cannot be entirely clear. Having said that, the interviews and observations allowed the unexamined – what experience means to these Sisters and how practice and experience move together – to be examined.

It seems that the Sisters concomitantly draw on experience and are adding to their experience whilst they work. Their everyday practices form the basis of their experience: they are also adding to their experience (and to their knowledge) whilst they are practising nursing (or going about their everyday activities at home, or in a classroom). The temporal nature of experience, its meaningfulness and its personal yet contextual nature, all contribute to its complexity and elusiveness.

Practising surgical nursing

The 'visible' form of the Sisters' experience can be found in their moment-by-moment work in the ward. The Sisters' central focus was helping the individual patient towards recovery and in order to do that they made the ward *work* for all the patients.

In their accounts of experiences with patients, the Sisters usually set situations or concerns within the framework of the patients' stay on the ward. This framework was reflected in daily practices. For example, at the change of shift handover reports, the nurses were told about the patients in relation to their stay in hospital. In contrast, the practices which make the ward work were organized around the workflow of a single shift.

Helping patients towards recovery

Many studies on patient recovery from surgery (cf. Seers, 1987; Wilson-Barnett and Fordham, 1982), in their concentration on the patient and recovery process, give the impression that patients recover from surgery with minimal nursing input. However, when the Sisters' experience is examined directly, a different view emerges. With their extensive repertoire of complex practices, the Sisters were seen to actively help patients through their surgical admission.

The Sisters recognized 'usual' patterns of recovery from their experience of many patients in similar situations. They linked their understanding of a particular patient's progress to what might be expected. However, it was impossible to extract from the Sisters' practice either rules for monitoring care or discrete phases of recovery. Their actual care of individual patients revealed a much more fluid and subtle, yet active process than is described in textbook treatments of preoperative and postoperative care. In the patients' postoperative stay in hospital, there were some notable ways in which the Sisters helped them towards recovery. One of these is in their careful vigilance and action.

Diligently watching

Upon the patients' return from the operating theatre, the Sisters began a period of closely monitoring individual aspects of the patients' physical status, including pulse, blood pressure, respirations, bleeding, pain, and in many cases, fluid balance. At the same time, they gathered a total picture or impression of the patient, including the significance of monitored signs. With experience, nurses become astute at picking up small changes in the patients' condition, what Benner (1984) terms 'graded qualitative distinctions'. The Sisters monitored each patient through the assigned nurses and focused selectively, 'keeping a close eye on' patients whose conditions were less stable.

In the following example, Sr Jarvis, with a first-year student, diligently watches a patient newly back from surgery, picking up the 'early warning signals' of postoperative bleeding following prostatectomy and acting on them. In contrast to a situation several years previously, where she only responded once the patient was in severe pain and the bladder clot had formed, Sr Jarvis now attends to more subtle signs of bleeding and acts much earlier, preventing the need for further surgery.

> Mr Scott was a gentleman who'd had a prostatectomy and he came back with bladder irrigation. Which was unusual because the consultant who'd operated normally . . . doesn't use irrigation. So I immediately thought that the reason for this must be that he'd had a large prostate resection. And his urine on return was really quite darkly haematuric.
>
> So I said to the student who was looking after him that she had to

be particularly careful at making sure his irrigation always ran fully on, so that there was no chance of it clotting off. And to keep a very close eye on his urine output. That it was very haematuric, more so than we would like. His blood pressure and pulse on return were comparable with his pre-op. But I told her to make sure she would let me know if it started to fall.

About an hour later she told me that his blood pressure had dropped by about 30 mm diastolic and so I then immediately increased his IV fluids. And phoned the resident . . . His blood pressure continued to drop and his urine still remained very haematuric so we started blood transfusions.

Following blood transfusions, the administration of atropine and about three hours of penile traction, the bleeding stopped and 'everything then went according to plan'.

In this situation, Sr Jarvis was alerted to the potential for bleeding because of a variation in the surgeon's usual post-operative procedure and confirmed it by the quality of haematuria: 'I wasn't happy with him from the minute he came back'. On the urology ward, the nurses recognized a range of haematuria and its significance in relation to normal progression or difficulties in recovery. In assessing the patient, and the significance of the clinical signs, Sr Jarvis included how the patient said he felt – 'he said he felt fine' – how he appeared, and when that changed: 'he initially looked fine . . . and just prior to the blood transfusion being started he looked to me quite pale. I noted he was a little bit clammy'. By understanding how quickly a patient's condition can change when he is bleeding, she alerted the student to the importance of 'diligently watching the patient from the minute they come back' and averted a more serious situation.

Recovery from the anaesthetic and the immediate effect of the operation takes from two to forty-eight hours for most patients. Barring complications, when the patient passes a turning point, 'the hump', the Sisters consider them to be 'on their way to recovery'. Diligent watching continues until the Sisters sense the patients are over the hump.

Making the ward work

In charge of a ward of twenty to thirty-six beds, the Sisters were responsible for ensuring the care of patients, managing the staff and material resources of the ward and contributing to the education of students. They were the coordinators and decision-makers at the centre of a complex, ever-changing network of communications, people and services (Runciman, 1983). They make their wards work in a way which enables them to achieve their goal of helping individual patients towards recovery (or to die peacefully).

The general tenor of the Sisters' experience and practices in making the ward work can be gathered through this example.

Keeping the workflow going with the patient at the centre

With a clear overview of the work to be done and the potential for each patient, the Sisters are able to combine actions, anticipate problems and coordinate activities, helping the nurses to achieve the goals of care for individual patients while addressing the needs of all. The Sisters have learned how to 'use every minute you have, and not to waste one second of a nurse's time'. This does not come easily, particularly when there is an ever increasing workload and too few people to help.

The Sisters talk about 'cutting corners' in such situations. 'Cutting corners' is not easily defined, but central to its meaning is being flexible and paring down actions. They are selective about which corners they cut and how they do it, not cutting corners to save time in the short run, when the long-term effect would be compromised recovery for a patient. On a very short-staffed day, Sr Calder gets Mr Thomas, an elderly patient with a fractured humerus and infected chest, sitting in a chair before breakfast so that his arm benefits from postural traction and he can breathe better. She not only sees the immediate task to be done, but has a broader plan for the patient and does what is necessary immediately to prevent complications later.

The Sisters recognize what would and would not be time saving, taking this broader goal into their definition of what may be minimum nursing care. Sr Calder describes how she sees the work organization in a different way from her staff nurses.

But they're not seeing it the same way as I see it . . . . Whereas they would see it – give him his breakfast in bed and then we'll be getting him up out of bed later – [to do his bath] . . . They would do breakfast first. They wouldn't see another job to do.

The Sisters understand their present actions as a part of a larger whole. They know where the patient is in the course of recovery, know where he has to get to and know what actions are required to get him there. It enables them to 'see another job to do'.

One of the several techniques used by the Sisters to keep the workflow going for patient care is to maximize the effect of their experience. Sometimes it means that the nurses become something of an extension of the Sisters. When Mr Scott needs 'diligent watching', Sr Jarvis is specifically directive. She could not count on the student's independent judgement and action.

And I felt it was up to me, not exactly to be looking after the patient on my own, but not relying on the nurse who was looking after the patient to pick up on the subtle changes that I was looking for.

The Sisters try to strike a balance between allowing the nurses independent action, while recognizing the needs of the patients and the nurses' limitations. As they give a report, help a student to get organized at a patient's bedside, or do a procedure they often say, 'the most important thing to remember is . . .'. In this way, the Sisters help the students attend to the most important concerns, concerns they would be attending to if they could be there.

In summary, the Sisters keep the work flowing through their own actions and by actively supporting others. They organize and coordinate the work and intervene where and when necessary to move it along. They continually revise priorities for care, keeping a finely-tuned tension between the needs of individual patients and the needs of the ward as a whole.

Noticing, understanding and acting

When the Sisters' everyday practices were examined more closely, a process of practising was discerned. This process, of noticing, understanding and acting, was evident in the relational and contextual nature of the Sisters' practices. Although noticing, understanding and acting can be differentiated conceptually, in practice they are not so neatly segmented. Rather, they are inextricably intertwined in a non-linear, non-sequential process. The qualitative character of this process seemed to contribute to the Sisters' practice being complex, multifaceted, goal-directed and centred on the patient.

Noticing is more than seeing, or hearing or assessing: it is a process of interpretation. Understanding is more than a surface knowing or recognition: it is a deep comprehension of meanings inherent in a situation. Acting goes beyond mere behaviour or deployment of skills: it is practising in a concrete situation (Figure 3.1).

Through their involved stance in the situation, the Sisters notice salient features, understand their meaning and act, making the ward work, caring for the patient. Sr Jarvis notices the bladder irrigation, understands it as a sign of potentially significant bleeding and acts, ensuring that Mr Scott is 'diligently watched'. Sr Calder notices Mr Thomas' posture, understands what it means in terms of his fracture, lung expansion and comfort in eating, and acts, getting him up for breakfast. In a handover report, Sr Baxter notices a student's 'wee delay' in responding to her suggestion that she take out a patient's central line. She understands the delay to be a lack of knowledge and confidence and she acts, arranging for the student to observe the procedure again. Noticing is made

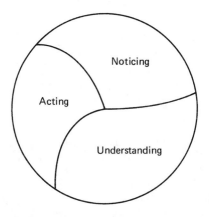

Figure 3.1 Noticing, understanding, acting

possible through the Sisters' experiences in previous, similar situations, which have made understanding possible.

Noticing and understanding are inextricably bound to the present context, as action occurs in an ongoing, concrete situation. Noticing and understanding are made possible by action. Sr Jarvis goes to see each patient returning from surgery and is frequently with junior nurses, checking to see how they are managing. Sr Calder, in the midst of the morning activities, is in a position to notice an opportunity for achieving several goals through getting a patient up for breakfast. Sr Baxter continually experiences being with students on the ward, understanding how they learn to do procedures and noticing what happens to the student and the patient when they are inadequately prepared. How the Sisters go about caring for patients through making the ward work is an active, interpretative process.

The Sisters also promote noticing in their interactions with students. With a patient who is bleeding postoperatively, Sr Jarvis advises the student about what to keep 'a very close eye' on. Sr Calder invites the students to compare similar responses of two patients to their different operations. Sr Inglis asks directly, 'He has a heparin pump. Do you know why?'. She goes on to tell about this patient's particular problems with anticoagulant regulation. The Sisters not only give factual information, they interpret the patients' conditions, advising junior nurses about the salient features of the patient and his situation. They help the junior nurses to learn how to notice, to pick up and to interpret.

In much of the Sisters' practice, it is impossible to identify practical know-how and theoretical knowledge separately. However, their theoretical knowledge becomes more apparent when they are teaching students. Knowledge of pressure and its practical implications informs Sr Grant's approach as she guides a student through the procedure of removing a central venous pressure catheter.

> Sr Grant goes to help Nurse Elias, a third-year student, to take out Mr Baker's CVP. Sr Grant tells Nurse Elias, 'If it is a positive CVP it means that the pressure in there (pointing to his chest) is less than the air. If the CVP is negative, the pressure of the air is greater. What position should he be in if it is negative, to avoid having an air embolism?' Nurse Elias: 'Sitting?' 'No, that would decrease the pressure in the chest'. Nurse Elias: 'Head further down'. 'Yes'. Sr

Grant then supervises as Nurse Elias takes it out. . . . As Nurse
Elias takes it out, Sr Grant says, 'Give it traction, steady traction,
pulling up . . .' Sr Grant repeats at the end of the procedure that
the most important thing to remember is to have Mr Baker in a flat
position.

Sr Grant did not go into the details of pressure in the chest, but
reminded Nurse Elias of the relationship of posture to pressure
and of the reading of the central line to air pressure. Although
theoretical principles informed her instruction, she focused on the
practical knowledge of the procedure. Sr Grant's understanding of
central lines and their removal was neither solely theoretical nor
practical. An admixture of theoretical knowledge and practical
know-how is evident in her practice.

The Sisters' practising, a process of noticing, understanding
and acting, is not an empty process, but one which is imbued with
knowledge and skills in specific situations.

Becoming experienced

A sense of the continuous interplay between experience and
practice clearly emerged from the Sisters' accounts and observations of their everyday practices. They were shown to be
'experienced' Sisters who were experiencing all the time. The
interconnection of experience and practice was revealed in the
process of practising: noticing, understanding and acting.

In talking about experience and learning Sr Inglis puts it simply
yet profoundly, 'It's happening all the time'. This almost
throw-away remark points towards the contextual and relational
nature of learning which arises out of experience itself. From this
study learning does not seem to be as discrete a phenomenon as
various experiential learning models (cf. Kolb, 1984; Boud,
Keogh and Walker, 1985) would suggest. Nor does learning seem
to be solely connected to reflection (cf. Schön, 1983).

Just as noticing, understanding and acting depict the process of
practising, so they could be taken to describe the process of
experiencing. Taking learning to depict the movement of
experiencing, it could be said that learning encompasses changes
in noticing, understanding and acting. In addition, learning is

made possible by noticing, understanding and acting. For the Sisters, becoming experienced surgical nurses seems to be a complex process, linked to their moment-by-moment practising.

It can be suggested that for the 'excellent, experienced' sisters in this study, being attuned to experience is at the centre of their everyday experience in practice. Being attuned to experience carries with it a sense of openness to experience, a dialogue with others and with oneself and an understanding of knowing which goes beyond theoretical knowledge.

Knowing in everyday practice

The Sisters' everyday practices would indicate that they are knowledgeable practitioners, continually deepening, refining and extending their knowledge by being attuned to experience. The knowledge they are extending in their everyday practice is, it could be suggested, knowing-in-practice.

Conventionally, knowledge and practice are understood to be two separate entities which may be joined or integrated. In common with other professions (Freidson, 1986; Clark, 1989), theoretical or informal knowledge is, with few exceptions, the most valued and recognized form of knowledge in nursing (Carper, 1978; Meleis, 1985). Practice, in the conventional view, is seen to be an arena of action or a separate behavioural world in which intentional actors use or apply knowledge. A prominent concern is to find ways in which theory and practice can be successfully integrated. The notion of using knowledge as a guide or base for practice provides perhaps, the unifying tie in the literature on the practice–theory connection.

Clark (1989) suggests that if theory is to be considered as being used or applied by practitioners, then it must be capable of clear explication and identified in practice. In this study of the Sisters' everyday experience it was impossible to discern knowledge or theory in an abstract form from observations of their practice, or from their accounts. But that does not mean that the Sisters do not have knowledge of theory or may not have originally learned some of their practice with the help of theoretical knowledge. Essentially, theoretical knowledge which they might once have had in the abstract form is no longer decontextualized and atemporal (timeless): it is embedded in the practical context. It has become part of knowing-in-practice. Indeed, theoretical knowledge is only visible in many situations because the Sisters are having to either explain or account for their practices. Even in these circumstances, knowing is seldom, if ever, expressed as isolated general theory. The knowing has its particular meaning because of the context.

Schön (1983, 1987) and Freidson (1986) both acknowledge the effect of the context of practice on the practitioner's knowledge. However, the inability to discern theoretical knowledge in the Sisters' practices suggests that Schön's (1987) argument that professionals operate from the basis of an interpersonal theory-in-use (that is the use of previously learned theory) is insufficient for explaining the configuration of knowing and practice in particular situations. The Sisters' practices did not appear to emanate from a theory, be it tacit or explicit. To suggest that they did negates the importance of the context in forming, and transforming, knowing.

Similarly, Freidson's (1986) suggestion that subjectively held theoretical knowledge is transformed into working knowledge is not evident. The separation of the knowing person and the world of practice was not found in this study. The Sisters' ongoing, taken-for-granted practices do not seem to be separate from themselves, nor separate from the specific context in which they are: their practices both form, and are formed by, the situation. Much of the time, the Sisters could not be said to 'hold' and 'use' knowledge: their knowing is already in their moment-by-moment practices.

The Sisters' knowing-in-practice has been found to be much like practical knowledge, which Dreyfus (1980) and Benner (Benner, 1984; Benner and Wrubel, 1989) suggest is the skilled know-how of everyday practical activity. However, theory is not absent from their practices. The Sisters' knowing-in-practice is imbued with theory and practical knowing. It is knowing in a context: theory cannot readily be discerned. Already a part of everyday, ongoing pragmatic activity and informed by theoretical knowing, knowing-in-practice is at the same time, more subtle and encompassing than the separate notions of practice and theory. Theoretical knowledge and practical knowing are already integrated in everyday practice.

Realizing the value of everyday experience

It has been suggested that the conventional distinctions of theory and practice were not evident in this study of the moment-by-moment, everyday experience of 'excellent, experienced' surgical ward sisters. When experience was directly examined it was found to be more complex and elusive than it is generally held to be. It is suggested that experience is inextricably bound with ongoing practices and, through them, with time. There is a continual interplay of the past, the present and the future in ongoing practising. It would appear that the Sisters become 'experienced' and develop expertise by being attuned to experience. Being attuned to experience is constituted by an inextricably intertwined process of noticing, understanding and acting which is made possible through a stance of involvement and care. The character of knowing, rather than being a use or application of theory in practice, is a more subtle distinction of knowing-in-practice.

It is tempting to try to extract what makes excellent, experienced nurses and sisters and place it between the pages of a textbook. This study has illustrated that, besides being impossible, such a course of action would be ill-advised. Nursing is about actively helping people to keep healthy and to care for people in times of illness. Learning to nurse well, it appears, occurs in milieux in which nurses are engaged in practice with patients and clients.

The insights gleaned from this study of excellent, experienced sisters spark a number of questions in this time of educational change prompted by Project 2000. Among them are:

- What is the nature of everyday experience to which students are attuned?
- How can learners be assisted to recognize similar aspects among different contexts, understand their meanings, make comparisons and connections, and have the confidence to act?
- How can the existing strengths of ward sisters' practices be enhanced?

It would seem opportune at this time, and in light of the findings of this study, to suggest a fundamental re-examination of the traditional distinctions of theory and practice. In the nursing literature, these distinctions not only apply to nursing knowledge, but also to the institutions and people who are concerned with teaching nursing and providing nursing care (cf. Miller, 1989). A fundamental re-examination is needed in order to raise new possibilities for advancing nursing care, education, research and administration. In order for these discussions to be successful in making a significant contribution to nursing, there must be adequate recognition of nurses' everyday experience.

References

Argyris, C. and Schön, D. (1974) *Theory in Practice: Increasing Professional Effectiveness*. Jossey Bass, San Francisco

Benner, P. (1984) *From Novice to Expert: Excellence and Power in Clinical Nursing Practice*. Addison-Wesley, California

Benner, P. and Wrubel, J. (1989) *The Primacy of Caring: Stress and Coping in Health and Illness*. Addison-Wesley, California

Boud, D., Keogh, R. and Walker, D. (1985) *Reflection: Turning Experience into Learning*. Kogan Page, London

Carper, B. A. (1978) Fundamental patterns of knowing in nursing. *Advances in Nursing Science*. 1, 13–23

Clark, C. L. (1989) Theory and Practice in Social Intervention: The Case of Voluntary Action on Unemployment. Unpublished PhD Thesis, University of Edinburgh

Diekelmann, N. (1988) From Layperson to Novice Nurse: The Lived Experiences of Nursing Students. Unpublished manuscript. Madison, Wisconsin: University of Wisconsin School of Nursing

Dreyfus, H. L. (1980) Holism and hermeneutics. *Review of Metaphysics*, 34, 3–23

Field, P. A. (1981) A phenomenological look at giving an injection. *Journal of Advanced Nursing*, 6, 291–296

Forrest, D. (1989) The experience of caring. *Journal of Advanced Nursing*, 14, 815–823

Freidson, E. (1986) *Professional Powers: A Study of the Institutionalization of Formal Knowledge*. University of Chicago Press, London

Gadamer, H-G. (1975) *Truth and Method*. Sheed and Ward, London

Gray-Snelgrove, R. (1982) The Experience of Giving Care to a Parent Dying of Cancer: Meanings Identified Through the Process of Shared Reflection. Unpublished PhD Thesis, Ontario Institute for Studies in Education, University of Toronto

Griffin, V. R. (1987) Naming the processes. In *Appreciating Adults Learning: From the Learners' Perspective* (eds D. Boud and V. Griffin), pp. 209–221. Kogan Page, London

Heidegger, M. (1962) *Being and Time* (translated by J. Macquarrie and E. Robinson). Basil Blackwood, Oxford

Henderson, V. (1966) *The Nature of Nursing*. Collier-Macmillan, London

Jarvis, P. (1987) *Adult Learning in the Social Context*. Croom Helm, London

Kitson, A. L. (1986) Indicators of quality in nursing care – an alternative approach. *Journal of Advanced Nursing*, 11, 133–144

Kitson, A. L. (1987) Raising standards of clinical practice – the fundamental issue of effective nursing practice. *Journal of Advanced Nursing*, 12, 321–329

Kolb, D. (1984) *Experiential Learning*. Prentice-Hall, Englewood Cliffs, New Jersey

Lathlean, J. (1987) *Job Sharing a Ward Sister's Post*. Ashdale Press, Peterborough

McFarlane, J. K. (1977) Developing a theory of nursing: the relation of theory to practice, education and research. *Journal of Advanced Nursing*, 2 (3), 261–270

MacLeod, M. L. P. (1990) Experience in Everyday Nursing Practice: A Study of 'Experienced' Surgical Ward Sisters. Unpublished PhD Thesis, University of Edinburgh

Magee, B. (ed) (1987) *The Great Philosophers*. BBC Books, London

Meleis, A. I. (1985) *Theoretical Nursing: Development and Progress*. J. B. Lippincott, Philadelphia

Meleis, A. I. (1987) ReVisions in knowledge development: a passion for substance. *Scholarly Inquiry for Nursing Practice: An International Journal*, 1 (1), 5–19

Melia, K. M. (1987) *Learning and Working: The Occupational Socialization of Nurses*. Tavistock Publications, London

Miller, A. (1989) Theory to practice: implementation in the clinical setting. In *Current Issues in Nursing* (eds M. Jolley and P. Allan). Chapman and Hall, London

Pembrey, S. (1980) *The Ward Sister – Key to Nursing*. Royal College of Nursing, London

Rabinow, P. and Sullivan, W. M. (1979) *Interpretive Social Science*. University of California Press, Berkeley

Ricoeur, P. (1979) The model of the text: meaningful action considered as text. In Rabinow, P. and Sullivan, W. M. (1979), *op. cit.*, pp. 73–101. (First published in *Social Research*, 38 (3), 1971)

Runciman, P. J. (1983) *Ward Sister at Work*. Churchill Livingstone, Edinburgh

Schön, D. A. (1983) *The Reflective Practitioner: How Professionals Think in Action*. Basic Books, New York

Schön, D. A. (1987) *Educating the Reflective Practitioner*. Jossey-Bass, San Francisco

Seers, C. J. (1987) Pain, Anxiety and Recovery in Patients Undergoing Surgery. Unpublished PhD Thesis, King's College, University of London

Smith, P. A. (1988) Quality of Nursing and the Ward as a Learning Environment for Student Nurses: A Multimethod Approach. Unpublished PhD Thesis, King's College, University of London

Strauss, A., Fagerhaugh, S., Suczek, B. and Wiener, C. (1985) *Social Organization of Medical Work*. University of Chicago Press, Chicago

Taylor, C. (1971) Interpretation and the sciences of man. *Review of Metaphysics*, 25 (1), 1–51. (Also in Taylor, C. (1985) *Philosophy and the Human Sciences. Philosophical Papers 2*. Cambridge University Press, Cambridge)

Thomas, A. M. (1986) Review of 'Adult learning: research and practice', by H. E. Long, *Learning* (Canadian Association for Adult Education), 4 (3), 21–22

United Kingdom Central Council (1987) *Project 2000: The Final Proposals. Project Paper 9*. United Kingdom Central Council for Nursing, Midwifery and Health Visiting, London

Wilson-Barnett, J. and Fordham, M. (1982) *Recovery from Illness*. John Wiley, Chichester

Part Two
Lecturer practitioners

When work started in the mid 1980s on a new programme for student nurses in Oxfordshire Health Authority a unique opportunity arose to explore radical ways of teaching practice. There had been a degree of dissatisfaction for some time over the division which occurred between classroom and clinical teaching, alongside a very strong commitment to the development of clinical nursing, coupled with organizational changes. Thus as the new curriculum emerged, work was also undertaken to develop new roles which would bring together the strengths inherent in teaching in both practice and lecture settings. The role which emerged was that of the lecturer practitioner which, in its purest form, vests the responsibility for the management of patient care and the teaching of students in one person.

At the time many people were anxious about whether or not the role could become a reality since the scope of responsibility was so wide. If it was to succeed there would have to be a radical review of the interrelationship of lecturer practitioners, not just with clinical teams with whom they would work, but also with the managers of the parent organization and the academic institution responsible for the students' educational programme. In other words there would be a need for a major cultural change within the whole organization in order to accommodate the change.

While it is widely recognized that one part of an organization cannot alter without having some impact on other parts, achieving change of this magnitude is no easy matter. The following three chapters offer some insight into the experience of three people who set out to respond to just this challenge.

As is always the way when new ideas are being explored not all lecturer practitioners have developed their roles in exactly the same way. The incumbents have been free to find approaches which are right for them as people and for the clinical settings in which they are working. This healthy variation is apparent in the way they have recalled their experiences.

Chapters 4 and 5 compliment one another in that they each describe one aspect of the development work which was undertaken. Thus in Chapter 4, Mary FitzGerald describes the first part of the story, covering critical work required at the beginning of a venture of this nature in developing the clinical area in which she was working. There is no doubt that this is an essential prerequisite to the creation of an effective learning environment for students but the impact on the quality of patient care does much to justify the time and energy needed for such changes.

Chapter 5, contributed by Sarah Burns, describes the way in which she addressed the second major component of the role, that is the creation of a clinically based teaching programme, tackling such issues as the assessment of clinical competence and the development of mentoring roles. It must, however, be stressed that the division between these two aspects of work is false and has only been presented in this way for convenience. In reality there was a strong interrelationship between the development of practice and the development of the teaching programme.

It has already been pointed out that there is no single right way of working as a lecturer practitioner and in Chapter 6, Ingrid Stevens offers a slightly different perspective although the principles of bringing together clinical and theoretical work remain the same. In this instance a collegiate model was developed with two people taking responsibility for different aspects of the work.

It is unlikely that all the ways in which people will work as lecturer practitioners in the future have been described here. However, the experiences described in the following three chapters offer valuable insights into some of the issues which need to be addressed and can act as a firm foundation for future developments.

4

Lecturer practitioner: creating the environment

Mary FitzGerald

Introduction

It is intended in this chapter to recall and explore my early work as a lecturer practitioner in an attempt to understand how both the role and the practice area in which I was working were developed. The first phase of the development, lasting nearly two years, was one of preparation. The initial broad aims were to develop and maintain a quality nursing service for clients, and thereby create an environment conducive to learning nursing. I was appointed as the lecturer practitioner to a twenty-bedded medical ward, two years before students from a new undergraduate nursing programme from the polytechnic would be placed there. Besides some curriculum development, teaching input to theoretical modules in the first year and some administrative work, the commitment to the polytechnic in the early days was light. This was intentional as it was generally recognized that the initial work of the lecturer practitioner would be concentrated on the service and the development of the clinical nursing team.

Critical examination of the experience may help to illuminate the path of others doing similar work. However, as the experience was, and remains, so particular to this specific ward and team of nurses no one could be expected to copy it precisely. It is not suggested, therefore, that the work could be generalized but that some important lessons can be gleaned from it.

The work in the initial phase was very difficult (FitzGerald, 1989a), but has now reached an extremely rewarding phase. It is possible that by recounting the early days some of the ideas may be influenced by the current state of optimism. A genuine attempt to recall the developments accurately has been made, but it is true that pain dims with time and is influenced by its productivity.

Since the role of lecturer practitioner was new, one of the first things I did was to write my own job description, which gave me some freedom to set priorities. I also had a well-developed strategy and ideas of the type of developments I wished to achieve in practice (FitzGerald, 1989a). These plans were influenced by my values, interests, and past clinical experience, which included years as a ward sister and nurse tutor. The 'District Philosophy of Nursing' and my own theoretical knowledge of nursing, management and teaching were also influential at this time.

The ward I was appointed to was an area I had worked in as a clinical practice development tutor. Before taking up post I had helped the nurses to formulate their views about ward philosophy. The content of this document emerged from their thoughts about the things they valued in nursing, but they had needed some assistance in writing down their ideas, which I was able to provide. It was helpful that the ward nurses already had this statement of beliefs and values before we started to work together, as much of the development work could be seen to stem from the shared philosophy rather than being the ideas of the new leader of the team.

Whilst working with the team on the philosophy, we had formed good relationships, so when some of the nurses asked me to apply for the vacant lecturer practitioner post I was delighted. Although it was not the best time for this career move I felt their support was too valuable to be missed. With hindsight, this was the correct decision, as someone coming in to make changes is in a difficult position. Getting the support and enthusiasm of the team who agree about fundamentals is indeed a head start (Wright, 1989).

Resources

Despite considerable knowledge and experience of the change process it is not surprising that this development did not assume classic lines. Pearson (1991) describes the notion of the 'chaos of practice' where the complexity and difficulties of nursing limit most espoused theory in use, and this was certainly our experience. Although I had intended to have a three-month assessment and settling phase this proved impossible. From the first day it was obvious that the ward had major problems mainly associated with inadequate staffing levels. I was immediately under pressure from two sources.

First, pressure came from the ward team. This was not overt but their strained faces, moans and dislike of the hospital nursing management were strong messages. Second, it came from senior nurses in the hospital. I was expected to take on immediate responsibility for the staffing numbers and to include myself in those numbers. Whilst most senior nurses in the hospital believed and expressed that the job was too much for one person to do, no one had any practical solutions or it seemed as if no one could offer any real help. I felt there was little enthusiasm for the new role and that I would be left to sink or swim alone. Of course there were other lecturer practitioners in the same boat, and their help and support was invaluable. In retrospect, there was little the other senior nurses could do to ease the situation. They, too, were overworked and demoralized after years of trying to provide a service which was inadequately resourced.

The problem of understaffing assumed huge proportions. It affected the standards of nursing practice on the ward, which at times did not meet the patients' physical needs. It seemed impossible that change could be achieved in this highly stressful environment. However, after a brief period of hysteria, I formulated a long- and short-term strategy, in the short-term filling in the shifts myself. Indeed, initially I worked more than five shifts per week which helped the immediate problem, and showed the team that their problems were mine too.

For a while I decided to put only one nurse on night duty. This strategy saved two nurses per week, for day duty. However, this put a strain on the night staff because they had to work each night with a nurse they did not know. I knew that help had to be sent to a single nurse on night duty whereas help was improbable in the day. This was an extremely unpopular decision with nurse managers and I was, quite rightly, called to account for it regularly. As soon as possible the night lines were covered again and have been consistently staffed for the last two years. A standard was written that there would always be two registered nurses on each shift. It was helpful for the staff to see how a standard of quality could work in their favour. When challenged about their need for staffing support from other areas in the hospital and the empty night lines, they quoted the standard and calmly asked if the other person disagreed with it. After the appointment of a new staff nurse, against much opposition from the rearguard of the old nursing management structure, this standard became a reality. The ward team could see that I had made a difference to their working lives. The team were beginning not only to accept but also to trust me.

As a longer term strategy it was decided to collect some empirical data to substantiate the case for a larger establishment. The nurses agreed to help record the data along with their subjective comments about the workload. This data, combined with two reports describing poor standards of care (FitzGerald, 1989a), were used to put the case to the unit accountant and other influential people in the district. In the first year *all* the medical wards had real increases in their nursing establishments; this achievement shows how work on a single unit can act as the trigger for wider change. The accountant sited the dependency data from my own and another lecturer practitioner's work when presenting the case of need. The ward repeated the dependency study annually for the following two years, and one of the staff nurses has now taken on the work as a longitudinal study for her dissertation.

There was also an element of luck. In the first year of appointment, the last junior students from the traditional school finished working on the ward and were replaced by staff nurses. These realistic replacement figures had been negotiated and worked out by nurses at district level, who understood the pressures nurses worked under and valued the nursing development which they believed would improve the nursing service offered to clients. That level of support was important. As can be imagined, having two staff nurses instead of two first-ward student nurses was indeed a boon to arranging and discharging nursing work.

I sought ways of improving the staffing levels of the ward at every opportunity. One year a charity grant was successfully applied for to pay for a part-time staff nurse to cover study leave for the nursing team. Nurses on post-basic courses, such as 'Care of the Elderly', and the 'Diploma in Nursing', were welcomed and offered clinical supervision in return for working with the team. As the ward's reputation improved and grew more opportunities of this sort arose.

In the early days I spent a lot of time working on the ward. This had its advantages as I got to know the rest of the team and they in turn began to feel comfortable with me. Nursing again after five years was both a trial and a joy. I had quite a lot to learn having been out of practice and being unfamiliar with the hospital. It was useful for the nurses to see that I really had a great deal to gain from them. However, it was also apparent to me that I had many skills that were immediately useful in the role – skills developed through a long nursing career and described by Watson (1985) as core skills, or things that good nurses do, no matter their location or medical speciality.

Other aspects of nursing which were more specific to the speciality had to be learnt, but this was stimulating. For example, finding out about the use of new drugs such as captopril and the care of someone starting this treatment, were essential to my role. What was distressing were the poor standards of care offered to patients on some shifts, coupled with physical tiredness and a feeling that I could not offer any more than I was in terms of time or effort. There were moments, when staffing was bad, that I despaired of the job. It is a dangerous time for a nurse when he or she has made the philosophical leap to new ways of nursing and yet cannot hope to meet those ideals in practice, for the levels of guilt and frustration can be very high. But this was exactly the path the whole team was going down. Thus, it was vital that the nursing establishment was increased and maintained for both the patients' and nurses' sakes.

Besides working with the staff I met with all members of the team on an individual basis, and gave them time to talk about themselves. I learnt of their aspirations, motivations and worries. Collectively the team planned to meet on a fortnightly basis. Initially I chose the agenda, although staff were invited to contribute to it and they always attended. However, subsequent reference to the minutes of these meetings seemed to indicate that they were not held as frequently as I recalled. The reason for this apparent discrepancy is that often the nurses decided they were too busy to stop work, and that sometimes minutes were not typed because I did not have time. It was not appropriate to delegate this work to the staff, because they saw themselves as overworked as it was, and were not wholly committed to the need for regular meetings. Now the staff arrange the meetings, take turns to be the chairperson, agree the agenda and write the minutes. I attend if possible but the team does not cancel or delay a meeting for me. It is my responsibility, just as any other member of the team, to read the minutes and make comment if necessary; however, it is clearly in my interests to get to as many meetings as possible.

In the early days I was wary of overloading the staff and did not delegate a great deal of work, although I intended to at a later date. The clinical regrading exercise of 1988 (a major reconstruction of clinical appointments which increased the number of clinical grades and awarded more money to nurses who accepted more responsibility) took place, and we were able to offer good grades to all the nurses. The three most experienced nurses were offered promotion in nine months if they fulfilled certain responsibilities. Gradually through this time they changed their work and status in the ward. They led teams of nurses, helped to select new team members, ensured adequate team cover, led discussions about patient care, wrote standards and took on specific responsibility for the ward learning environment, day-to-day management and clinical standard setting and monitoring. It would have been difficult to give them these responsibilities permanently if I could not offer suitable remuneration.

So before introducing change to nursing practice I tried to solve the problems associated with understaffing, attempting to get to know the staff and to feel an accepted member of the team whilst at the same time practising and regaining skills as a nurse. I felt it was important not to undermine the work the team was already doing with change that was premature.

Whilst these events may sound disjointed, it was practical to seize any opportunity that occurred. This sometimes led us down an unplanned path. There was not a grand plan, but it was important to realize that a great deal of thought went into all the development, and I spent a long time thinking about the ward. New work and change were often generated as opportunities arose. For example, the development of the team leader roles, and their ability eventually to take delegated responsibilities for managing their teams and some aspects of ward work, was not apparent when I accepted the lecturer practitioner position. Seeing potential gain from situations, and capitalizing on them, was far more effective than sticking to any rigid plan, however well-thought through it had been.

Introducing change

In reality the nurses were itching to change practice. They had been uncomfortable with the work organization on the ward since they had written their philosophy, which stated they believed in continuity of care for patients. At the time nurses were assigned to work at one or other end of the ward. As one end tended to be 'heavier' than the other they would swop over the next day. This arrangement meant that they did not often look after a patient for two days in a row.

They had expected me to come as a change agent and did not understand the delay. Whilst I was on holiday the team made a decision to change to team nursing. It was well organized and running relatively smoothly on my return. Whilst I was surprised by their independence and perceived prematurity in instigating this development, on the whole I was pleased that they felt confident enough in their own ability to make decisions without me. It would appear that I had been unduly wary about introducing change too quickly. Indeed Manthey (1980) sees no need for protracted preparation for primary nursing, and Ottoway (1976) advocates that education should follow change. I would challenge both views, but they were borne out in this instance. Team nursing made such a difference to our practice. We began to relate to patients we looked after each day. We began to discuss the course of nursing care within the team and sought information regarding certain patient problems. It was then possible to introduce other changes.

It was at this time that the concepts identified in the philosophy, in idealistic terms, became possibilities in practice. We started to clarify what we meant by notions such as partnership, advocate, caring and research-based practice. There were many sources for our learning – past experience, discussion, debate and literature. As time progressed we modified our practice to correspond with more sophisticated ideas. For example, we changed the terminology we used and described problems which were patient-centred. In order to give patients more opportunity to be involved in their care, we began to give a handover report at the bedside once a day. Assessments and care plans were written with the patients, and they were encouraged to share them with their partners or family if they thought it appropriate. Issues such as confidentiality, advocacy and locus of control were discussed with the team. These changes were motivated by our new understanding of partnership, and later, empowerment for patients.

Orem's (1980) conceptual model for nursing had been chosen by the ward team and was gradually introduced into practice. Instead of changing the documentation, the team looked at their practice and tried to identify systems of care, such as supportive, educative or wholly compensatory approaches, and choose appropriate nursing and client actions. Gradually we tried to work in partnership with patients and families by sharing nursing notes and including families and friends into the plan whenever appropriate.

Literature reviews for topics we found interesting and which were pertinent to our practice were gradually compiled. A review of the literature related to temperature taking and recording, patient education, near-death experiences, intravenous cannulation and mouth care were a few examples. Sometimes the work was used to justify a change in practice or the establishment of a clinical standard. This work was usually, but not always, completed because it was an official part of the Primary Nursing Module, an educational course run locally in preparation for practice as a primary nurse. Nurses who contracted with me for time to go on this course agreed to finish the assignment work, and to share new knowledge with the rest of the team. Other members of the team took an interest in the topic chosen for the literature review.

There was some resistance to intellectual enquiry before change, demonstrated by the premature move to team nursing, and a reported comment from one of the staff nurses when someone proposed a change – 'don't ask her, you'll have to write a paper!'. I was aware of the rumblings and acknowledged the difficulty people had studying after a long day and tried not to make staff feel they had to do more work. However, I continued to encourage nurses at what I hoped were appropriate times. I bargained over study leave, and on the whole the staff gave back twice as much time in project work as they had in study time. I included nurses in outside teaching work, such as primary nursing visitor days and reflective practice lectures, as they were becoming increasingly conversant in both subjects. This work was a great motivator for us to read and learn.

The change to primary nursing was more controlled than that to team nursing. All the staff wanted to change to primary nursing and it was a long-term goal from the start. There were various motives for this. Primary nursing was currently fashionable in the United Kingdom and wards using it had high status and profile – one nurse was heard to say it would look good on her CV. The nurses also wanted to have their own defined areas of responsibility and to be able to see results of their own work. They saw primary nursing as a system that would help them to put their philosophy of nursing into practice. I shared the staff nurses' motives but had other vested interests. Primary nursing would further devolve responsibility for patient care to the staff, thus freeing up my time. Primary nurses had to be knowledgeable in order to prescribe nursing care for which they were accountable. These 'knowledgeable practitioners' would be mentors to the polytechnic undergraduates who were starting in eighteen months.

The nurses themselves proposed who should be primary nurses when the system eventually changed. This in fact was made easier by the regrading programme. I proposed a structure with more primary nurses with low case loads, rather than the one adopted in other parts of the hospital where there were only three primary nurses, all at the most senior staff nurse grade on the ward. I felt this was right for two reasons. First, it was important for morale in order to make all the nurses feel they were involved in the change. They needed to see that their hard work was appreciated and that they were trusted to be or become primary nurses. Second, I wanted primary nurses to have smaller case loads so that they could concentrate on developing relationships with the patients and their families, and improve their decision-making skills.

A series of study days were designed, and the staff attended them in threes. The principles of primary nursing were discussed and new job descriptions examined thoroughly. I drew up a learning contract with each nurse, identifying progress that needed to be made in order to fill a role in the new system. Some choices of work were: to complete an in-house learning package which introduced students to Orem's model; to read *The Practice of Primary Nursing* (Manthey, 1980); to attend the 'People Skills course' which was offered locally; to have three successful audits of their care plans done and so forth. At a ward meeting it was decided that we would change to primary nursing when all the contract work was completed. The majority of work was completed two months later than planned, and in honesty not all was done. Nevertheless, the move was made at a time when the staff felt ready.

The change to primary nursing was quite easy. The team structure was maintained. Within the teams the nurses had already adopted patients with whom they always worked when on duty, and their knowledge and experience increased, so they were able to offer more to these patients. The relationship was now formalized through primary nursing and communicated to others in a range of ways. A white board in the centre of the ward, and the primary nurse's name on the front of the patient's nursing folder were introduced. Changes to the role of the coordinator, which always used to be held by the senior nurse on duty, occurred slowly until now there is little for the coordinator to do besides checking the emergency equipment and liaising with admissions, neither a high status nor a particularly popular job. Doctors' rounds were a problem for a long time and the primary cause of concern for the medical staff. Eventually one of the consultants suggested that the nurses draw up a list of order of the round. Now one nurse starts the round and sees all his or her patients and then finds the next nurse. This flexibility on the medical staff side has made a great difference to the quality of the nursing input to the rounds. It is suspected that it would not have been suggested if the work of the primary and associate nurses was not valued.

Quality assurance

Establishing and monitoring the quality of the nursing service was an essential part of my work. Three quality assurance tools have been used since the beginning. Yearly QUALPAC (Wandelt and Ager, 1974) assessments are made, which look at the quality of nursing, and the scores have risen steadily. The reports give information to the team about the different aspects of their practice. Mindful of some of the disadvantages of QUALPAC, the team appreciate this feedback and have always used the report to address problems and pay attention to practice as others see it. The Clinical Learning Environment Assessment Tool (Spouse, 1990) is also used once a year. This is carried out by an independent practitioner and nurse tutor, and the scores for this have remained consistently high. The nursing care plans are audited (Bayntun-Lees, 1988) regularly by the nurses on the ward, three being reviewed every three months.

An attitude that has been fostered amongst the nursing team, and which has been important in terms of maintaining standards, is an understanding of the usefulness of criticism and frank feedback between team members. It is acceptable to question other people's work and to ask them to change if this can be justified. This is not always achieved without personal pain, but other members of the team accept the behaviour and support both parties. It is now considered unhealthy to criticize a colleague's professional expertise covertly. If there is a problem it is considered carefully and then dealt with.

Some standards of performance (FitzGerald, 1989a; Robinson and FitzGerald, 1990) were written. These were particularly useful at the time when the team was considering roles and responsibilities. Clinical standards usually emanated from a clinical problem. For example, a small number of patients had developed phlebitis around their intravenous infusion sites, so a standard was written for the care of a patient with an intravenous cannula in position. It was far more difficult to write standards for more complex treatments, like aromatherapy, and in these areas the work was slower.

Each year I write a review of work achieved and in progress. This is submitted to another lecturer practitioner who validates the content by working with me and visiting the clinical area. The review is sent to the Head of the Polytechnic Department and the Director of Nursing Services. It is also sent for information to various strategic people such as the chief nurse, the consultants, and the district and unit general managers. It is politically useful for lecturer practitioners if others know what good work is being done. I also welcome feedback from the ward team about my work and accept comment from the lecturer practitioner who validates my review. I do not expect a great deal of feedback from the Head of the Department nor the Director of Nursing Services because they rarely see my work first hand. Rather this review is an opportunity for me to demonstrate the developments which are occurring in practice. This method of appraisal gives the appraisee much more control than old systems where results depended to a great extent on the appraiser's subjective judgement. If the days of short-term contracts and performance-related pay are coming, it could be that employees would feel more confident with this type of scheme.

Staff appraisal is an area that has not taken off in quite the way intended. Originally I planned that the staff would write standards of performance related to their job descriptions (FitzGerald, 1989b). Although the work started, not enough standards were written. It proved to be time consuming and there were always other things that needed to be done. The staff have had easy access to me, and it has been a priority to find time for someone who needs it. Nurses are encouraged to estimate their own progress and discuss it with either a team leader or me. However, formal feedback in the form of a written appraisal has not been done regularly. This is regretted by all of us, and in the future it is planned to adopt a system similar to the one I have used myself. The staff will write their profiles with help and supervision from more experienced colleagues and present them to the team. This will fit in neatly with the recommendations made by the United Kingdom Central Council (1990) in relation to professional profiling.

Educational opportunities taken by the nurses have ranged from accredited courses to days off to think. The ward has a higher than average amount of study leave recorded. The library on the ward has been added to consistently over the years, and staff regularly lend or borrow each others' books.

I have not managed to do any formal research since an early action research project (FitzGerald, 1989a). However, each year one clinical research project is launched. For example, a staff nurse did a small study into nurses' perceptions of their role as health educators (Dudley, 1991) and this work has been incorporated into practice. Another study is an examination of assessment, and it is hoped that this project will lead to a doctoral thesis.

By increasing responsibility and educational opportunities at the same time as making organizational changes, the nurses on the ward have become empowered. They have a great deal of confidence when working and know what they can do without asking permission. This process required a raising of consciousness which started before I took up post as lecturer practitioner, when the philosophy was written. For example, in the early days staff would ask if they could go home early. They were always answered 'I don't know . . . can you?'. They soon learnt that I did not want to make all the decisions for them. The only requirement was that a decision-maker could account for his or her choice. As the work organization changed to primary nursing each nurses' responsibility became clearer. It was easier to calculate one's workload and plan to come late to work or go early. In reality the nurses all worked more hours than they should have, and of course irregular hours had to be agreed with the rest of the team.

The changes made by the team were informed by theory. Personally I had been impressed by the work of Pearson (1983, 1988), Wright (1986, 1989) and Binnie (1987, 1988), all British nurses who have put considerable thought into changing nursing practice. The team were encouraged to read these works along with that of some of the American nurse theorists, notably Manthey (1980), Watson (1985), Styles (1983), Benner (1984) and Benner and Wrubel (1989). Whilst the ideas of these authors have not been used as blueprints for the nursing development, their work has increased the team's repertoire of nursing knowledge, and has helped team members to formulate plans and solve problems in their particular context and circumstances.

I am aware that all the developments have been a team effort. I am delighted that my original notion that most nurses, given more responsibility at a measured pace and accompanied with the right amount of challenge and support, are capable of working as autonomous professional practitioners (FitzGerald, 1990). The achievements of the nurses, both collectively and individually, are impressive, as evidenced by their publications (Dudley, 1991; Robinson and FitzGerald, 1990; Loader, 1990; Cabell, 1990; Garbett, 1990), prizes and scholarships and the obvious respect they have from other professionals (Northcott, 1991).

Although the team's contribution is acknowledged, the role of the lecturer practitioner as a change agent cannot be denied. Whilst I encouraged a democratic decision-making process, I was quite aware that my knowledge and ability to argue my point convincingly allowed me to manipulate the course of events to a certain extent. Wright (1989) stresses the importance of a change agent with advanced knowledge. As the nurses developed and became used to the open atmosphere, where constructive criticism and argument is appreciated, this manipulation became less obvious and would be less effective now as the staff have become more personally empowered.

It would be interesting to see how the team behave when I eventually leave. Indeed, they do manage quite well without me for fairly long periods especially during term time. However, when several nurses left the ward, followed by a period of understaffing, I was used in a more conventional way. It seemed that all problems were referred to me again; stress levels rose and to some extent these were transferred to me. This is an interesting observation which suggests that all developments should be constantly worked at to be maintained. It also highlights the continuing requirement for strong clinical leadership. The ward is a dynamic system that can easily progress or regress, a notion that all staff need to be aware of.

In summary, the achievements have been hard earned and development work is still required, especially in relation to patient satisfaction measurement. However, the ward has become an area that is conducive to learning, a view substantiated by early student evaluations. Nurses can demonstrate nursing practice that is worthy of critical analysis and students feel safe to practice and learn nursing. The staff are confident mentors who welcome questions and enjoy working with nursing students and patients. This learning environment has been achieved by concentrating on nursing practice, and the development of individual nurses.

It is my opinion that this type of work can be undertaken and maintained most successfully by an internal change agent, someone who has the status, power and authority of a ward sister/charge nurse. With this status I have been at liberty to empower the staff to bring about and maintain change.

The lecturer practitioner who is both lecturer and ward charge nurse, or practice area leader, is indeed stretched, especially in the early days of development. However, the control does make life easier. It is in areas where change is needed that this type of lecturer practitioner is most appropriate.

Mary FitzGerald has left the ward since this chapter was written and is now studying full-time for a doctoral thesis in Australia. We are pleased to report that the changes in practice have been sustained and indeed are still moving forward.

References

Bayntun-Lees, D. (1988) Care plan audit. In *A Systematic Approach to Nursing Care*, 2nd edn (Open University, Department of Health and Welfare). Open University Press, Buckingham

Benner, P. (1984) *From Novice to Expert*. Addison-Wesley, California

Benner, P. and Wrubel, J. (1989) *The Primacy of Caring: Stress and Coping in Health and Illness*. Addison-Wesley, California

Binnie, A. (1987) Primary nursing – structural changes. *Nursing Times*, 83 (39), 36–37

Binnie, A. (1988) The Working Lives of Staff Nurse: A Sociological Perspective. Unpublished MA Thesis, Warwick University

Cabell, C. (1990) Regaining a basic pleasure. *Nursing Times*, 86 (47), 27–29

Dudley, A. (1991) Different approaches to educating patients. *Nursing Times*, 87 (19), 44

FitzGerald, M. (1989a) Lecturer Practitioner: Action Researcher. Unpublished MN Thesis, University of Wales, Cardiff

FitzGerald, M. (1989b) Performance planning and review. In *Managing Nursing Work* (eds B. Vaughan and M. Pillmoor). Scutari Press, London

FitzGerald, M. (1990) Autonomy for practising nurses. *Surgical Nurse*, 3 (6), 24–26

Garbett, R. (1990) Patient Assessment in Primary Nursing. Unpublished BN Dissertation, University of Wales, Cardiff

Loader, S. (1990) Heaven can wait: near death experiences. *Professional Nurse*, 5 (9), 458, 460, 462–463

Manthey, M. (1980) *The Practice of Primary Nursing*. Blackwell Scientific, Boston

Northcott, N. (1991) Getting back to my roots. *Nursing*, 4 (31), 29–30

Ottoway, R. (1976) A change strategy to implement new norms, new styles and new environment to the work situation. *Personnel Review*, 5 (1), 13–18

Orem, D. (1980) *Nursing: Concepts of Practice*, 2nd Edn. McGraw-Hill, New York

Pearson, A. (1983) *The Clinical Nursing Unit*. Heinemann, London

Pearson, A. (1988) (Ed) *Primary Nursing: Nursing in the Burford and Oxford Development Units*. Croom Helm, London

Pearson, A. (1991) *Changing the Patterns of Nursing Care*. 6th National Conference for Ward Sisters, Kensington Town Hall, London, 15–16 April

Robinson, K. and FitzGerald, M. (1990) Setting ward standards. *Nursing Times*, **86**(14), 42–43

Spouse, J. (1990) *An Ethos for Learning*. Scutari Press, London

Styles, M. (1983) *On Nursing: Towards a New Endowment*. C. V. Mosby, St Louis

United Kingdom Central Council for Nursing, Midwifery and Health Visiting (1990) *The Report of the Post-Registration Education and Practice Project*. UKCC, London

Watson, J. (1985) *Nursing: The Philosophy and Science of Caring*. Colorado Associated University Press, Colorado

Wright, S. (1986) *Building and Using a Model of Nursing*. Edward Arnold, London

Wright, S. (1989) *Changing Nursing Practice*. Edward Arnold, London

Wandelt, M. and Ager, J. (1974) *Quality Patient Care Scale*. Appleton-Century-Crofts, New York

5

Lecturer practitioner: the reality of students

Sarah Burns

Introduction

The role of a lecturer practitioner has many aspects including clinical work, management, staff development, education and research. All are important, but inevitably there will be a different emphasis on the different parts of the job over time. This is especially so when the role is part of a new nursing structure in a health authority, and a critical component of a newly implemented and evolving programme of nurse education. Chapter 4 described how one lecturer practitioner spent the first two years following appointment immersing herself in all facets of the job, but concentrating in particular on the development of practice, her clinical area and her staff. This chapter focuses on the way in which student nurses influence life in the ward.

The clinical context for my lecturer practitioner role is a two-ward surgical unit. As lecturer practitioner I am senior nurse for the unit as well as sister to one of the wards. Primary nursing within a team structure is practised in the unit, and at the time of writing I have been in post for three years.

My intention is to explore the implications of nursing students on clinical placement in the unit for lecturer practitioners. However, as a starting point it would be helpful to give some background information to this placement, including a description of the student programme and in particular the practice modules which lead to a nursing degree.

The undergraduate programme is modular in structure: half the modules which students undertake are 'practice' and half are 'theory'. All modules are graded and the marks contribute to the overall honours degree classification. The students are placed with the lecturer practitioners to complete their practice modules. However, the day-to-day supervision of the students in practice is undertaken by mentors.

Perhaps the first thing to say is that there is a distinct feel to term and non-term time. Therefore, one can deduce that the students on placement do have an impact. But what is the impact and how are issues raised being handled? Four areas for discussion will be addressed:

- Role, preparation and support of mentors when students are on placement.
- Assessment of competence and awarding of grades for practice.
- The organizational issues and consequential reprioritizing of work for the lecturer practitioner.
- Areas for further work.

Role, preparation and support of mentors

It is apparent when looking at the nature of the work of lecturer practitioners and the numbers of students on placement for practice modules, that student contact and direct one-to-one clinical time must be limited. However, the philosophy of the undergraduate programme indicates that close personal supervision and negotiation of individual learning needs for nursing students are important. As it would not be possible for the lecturer practitioner to do all this, someone else must be identified, and this is where the mentors come into play.

The role of mentor

Mentors have been used in nursing education before, and support for the role is endorsed by the profession's regulating bodies (English National Board, 1987). While the profession itself agonizes over the pros and cons of mentors in educational situations (Ogier, 1987; Kershaw, 1990; Morle, 1990), for pragmatic reasons lecturer practitioners need someone to function as clinical supervisor and mentor for individual students when on clinical placement.

The nursing literature comments on the conflict anticipated in asking mentors to both supervise and assess students' competence. The English National Board condones the duality of role in mentoring (Fardell, 1988; Foy and Waltho, 1989), but critics comment that the mentoring component described in many definitions is at variance with the assessment role. It can be argued, however, that in this situation 'assessment' is too strong a word with disciplinary overtones, whereas 'giving constructive criticism' is perhaps more accurate and acceptable. Semantics matter in nursing. Anyone introducing change knows how sensitive nurses are to the words and phrases used to describe nursing activities. It would seem that the use of the term 'constructive criticism' within a nurturing relationship maybe more appropriate. This is the sense in which the mentor assesses.

A further argument as to why mentors are best placed to assess competence arises from the fact they are practice-based. Assessment of clinical competence by people who are not current in clinical practice is not justifiable in nursing today. The appreciation and understanding of the clinical context in which the nursing student is working is vital for sound constructive criticism. The 'messiness' of practice – it is not exactly as described in the text book – and the uniqueness of each patient's or client's needs has to be acknowledged when helping nursing students develop the ability to problem-solve clinical issues. It seems obvious that it is the practitioner working with the student who is the most appropriate person to assess. The mentor is well able and expected to use her professional judgement in this matter. Indeed, it can be suggested that this is a clear professional responsibility, in that there is an expectation of all members of the profession to be involved in the development and education of new nurses.

With these responsibilities of mentors clarified, the working definition of mentoring becomes clearer. A mentor may be defined as follows: 'a competent practitioner who facilitates a student's clinical learning within a one-to-one relationship, supervising and validating competency'.

It is perhaps worth commenting on the use and implications of the word 'competent' in this context. Benner (1984) distinguishes between a competent practitioner, as someone who still operates from rules or guidelines, and an expert practitioner who often works intuitively, using tacit knowledge, and jumping from stage to stage with little or no apparent logic. Further, the expert practitioner may have difficulty articulating her expertise since intuition is often difficult to analyse. Therefore, it could be argued that the nursing student, especially at the beginning of his or her programme and process of learning, would gain more from having a so-called competent practitioner as a mentor, rather than one deemed to be an expert. Then at a later stage, when the student is engaged in advanced practice and has more experience of making sense of things, an expert practitioner could be more appropriate. This seems to be supported by the view expressed by some students who initially see the staff nurses to be 'more at [their] level' than the lecturer practitioner, whereas later, when they – the students – are more confident about their knowledge and ability to reflect, the lecturer practitioner or the more senior ward nurses are seen as the people who can take them on further in their understanding of practice.

In terms of the relationship of students to mentors, the students are entirely supernumerary while on practice modules. Their clinical days are determined by individual module timetabling and as a consequence there is a marked level of negotiation between students and mentors about clinical time. Students can and do work weekends in order to work with their mentor. This also provides an extended clinical period where it is possible for students to see the impact of continuity of care and to participate in it.

Mentors function as individual clinical supervisors of students, particularly with first- and second-year students, where clinical competence is in its early stages of development. For safety reasons the student is only on duty when the mentor is.

Preparation

A key feature to surviving life as a lecturer practitioner is having confidence in the quality of work undertaken by mentors. Mentor preparation is entirely the responsibility of the lecturer practitioner. It is, therefore, an important part of her work, and it facilitates the development of a close relationship and a thorough understanding of the mutual roles between both parties. The formal preparation mainly comprises two-day courses run by small groups of lecturer practitioners, during which the role of the mentor and an outline of the programme are discussed. In the early days no qualified nurse had experienced the programme so we all had to make the effort to try and see how it might feel from the students' point of view. The specific learning focus for the students in the placement is explored in order that the mentors know what the students should be trying to get to grips with. For example, in our case they are studying the needs of the acutely ill patient, the adult with health disorders and their nursing care.

During the course the purpose of the mentor's role is discussed. Specific ward objectives, with ticks being placed on pieces of paper indicating that a task has been done, are not the order of the day. Rather, the mentor supports and challenges on an individual basis the objectives identified by the student, and subsequently negotiates learning needs. Daloz (1986) suggests that by defining and giving detail to supportive and challenging behaviours, mentors derive a clearer understanding of their role, gaining a vision or picture of the end point which can in turn be visualized and achieved by the student.

Support

The reality is that while students are on placement mentors themselves require support and guidance as they deal with their responsibilities. To this end, mentors have asked for support meetings to be held regularly, and while there is increasing familiarity with the processes involved in mentoring, new mentors find the support meetings especially useful. As a lecturer practitioner I may become involved in helping resolve particular issues, employing brainstorming strategies to resolve problems such as student distress in response to observed care, or dealing with criticisms by nursing students of other disciplines, for example, discussing doctors' ward round behaviours and quality of interpersonal skills. We have found that the open discussion of issues as they arise allows for a 'pot pourri' of other possible solutions to be generated. The following example illustrates the point.

The student, who was gaining her first clinical experience in my clinical area, expressed an interest in finding out more about what went on in the operating theatre. She wanted to be more informed when talking with patients and staff, so she went to observe a major operation being carried out on one of the patients from the ward. However, she had to leave the theatre before the operation was completed as she had a seminar to attend, so she did not see the end of the operation nor the patient's recovery of consciousness from anaesthetic.

Half way through the seminar that afternoon she felt herself switching off and thinking about what she had observed that morning. She noted the handling of the unconscious patient as being different – that everyday conversations continued over the patient and that the staff seemed not to acknowledge the patient. It was striking for her that the patient was not contributing. The goriness of the situation was not upsetting, as might have been expected, but the handling of the patient and his insides seemed reminiscent to her of a butcher's block.

As she left the seminar she bumped into a friend. They swapped stories of their experiences and as she described her own she burst into tears. She was distressed that this experience had generated such an emotional response – what was wrong with her?

The student wrote about this incident in her reflective diary, and when reviewing her learning contract with her mentor it was discussed. Her mentor acknowledged and confirmed that it was alright not only to feel but to express these feelings. The mentor was allowing freedom of expression, not judging or feeling threatened or defensive that there may be criticism of care within the experience described. The mentor went on to ask further questions about the experience, asking the student to explore other perspectives of the situation. The questions posed by no means dismissed the experience but helped the student gain a more rounded picture. Such explorations may identify for her a shortfall of knowledge about the situation. It may illuminate previously unconsidered points of view. It allows for a measured and considered opinion of the situation – in this case the implications of leaving the operation before its completion, and her feelings of incompleteness which may distort her picture. It allows for objectivity to be applied to a subjective experience.

The impact of the first witnessing of surgery was included in two other nursing students' learning contracts. The details were different but the core of the problem was the same. The mentor support group discussed the whole issue. We examined the pros and cons of theatre visits, and came to the conclusion that the first visit was one where the students felt very much at sea and were unable to make sense of the experience by themselves. Theatre staff, while friendly and open, were doing their work and were unable to pick up the students' anxieties. This was partly because the students were unable to articulate them well and partly because the theatre staff did not know the students and were unable to anticipate individual anxieties. The mentors came to the conclusion that if students were to observe their first operation, specific learning objectives should be teased out beforehand and some preparatory discussion should take place to try and identify likely stressors. Recently not all students have felt they wanted to go to theatre. We seem to have lost the 'tick it off' mentality and those who have wanted to have had particular reasons and usually go with their mentors. Thus it would seem that in encouraging the reflection of distressing experiences for students, and by exploring the whole, we have been able to learn ourselves and gain some idea of how best to support and challenge students in the process.

Mentorship and staff development

The first advantage of preparing mentors in my own clinical area is that I can combine the need for individual staff development with that of mentor development. This concept is important. When I can be confident about the quality of mentoring then control of the job is a reality. In my situation, though immediate clinical supervision has been delegated, control of the ethos and approach to care has been retained.

A second feature is that personal knowledge of mentors allows for effective feedback to be given to them on the quality of their work in this area, as well as being able to tailor mentor to students and vice versa. Another beneficial effect is that since I know the work of primary and associate nurses I am aware of the extra work I am asking these nurses to take on in relation to mentoring. While financial reward is not a reality, time back in lieu and real appreciation of the effort expended is well received by the mentors, and further enhances the lecturer practitioner's credibility within the clinical area. Thus, a problem that sometimes arises when nurse teachers are perceived to be unaware of the workload implications of asking trained staff to supervise clinical learning, is overcome.

In conclusion, preparation and support of mentors is an important part of my work. However, it neatly combines with staff development and monitoring of standards of clinical care, and provides learning opportunities for all the team.

Assessing competence and grading practice

The philosophy of the undergraduate course states that the ability to practise nursing is as important as understanding the theory of nursing. Fifty per cent of the modules are practice modules, and the classification of the degree gained is determined by grades achieved in *all* modules. Thus practice has to be graded just as essays and theoretical work are.

Part of my job as a lecturer practitioner is to grade practice module work. This is achieved in the following way. First, the criteria for grading are explicit and agreed by all teaching staff, and are presented in clear terms for all involved – students, mentors, lecturer practitioners, and lecturers.

Second, students complete written learning contracts giving evidence of clinical experience which demonstrate competency achievement. The choice of experiences and the presentation of the evidence is their responsibility, but discussion with mentors is important. The mentors are asked to validate the clinical experiences offered in the contract.

The third aspect of grading is the student's self-assessment. Confirmation of grade is given in discussion with the mentor and lecturer practitioner during a viva interview. In effect a triumvirate is convened to decide on the grade. It is important to note that while the formal grading process is carried out at the end of the module, the learning contract is a dynamic tool which is used throughout the placement, and informally the student is aware of the level of work she or he is achieving.

In order to ensure that there is consistency of grading across lecturer practitioners, moderation of learning contracts is carried out by all the module team at the end of the module. This process involves confirmation of consistency of grading in a double marking process, followed by review of work in all the different grades, to ensure consistency within the grade bands. It has been remarkably reassuring to note the agreement over grading, particularly where there has been cross-field marking, for example, between general and mental health or learning disability nursing.

The grading process, as indicated earlier, is the responsibility of the lecturer practitioner. The grading interviews with students and mentors at the end of placement take at least an hour. This interview is used to explore some of the contract content, to validate the competency achievement suggested by the student and explore the real level of understanding the student has. It is also an opportunity for the mentor to give further information to support the contract and to put forward any extenuating circumstances that have influenced the quality of the contract. With up to six students on placement at a time it can get quite busy fitting these interviews in at the end of term, especially as they often coincide with other marking activities. Inevitably this can have an impact on my being able to undertake clinical work at the same time.

Grading criteria are explicit and documented for all involved. Students are required to achieve competencies – as outlined in the handbook – within modules. The students refer to the competencies to help them identify their learning objectives, and use them when reflecting on clinical experiences and trying to make sense of what they have been involved in. Throughout all this they can, and do, use their mentor when reflecting. The grading profiles are also explicit and detail is given about what constitutes each different grade. Figure 5. 1 provides extracts from actual learning contracts.

In these examples the grading process becomes clearer. The evidence is there (or not) for grading. However, other issues have arisen which need exploring. First, there may be some confusion regarding whether grading involves the assessment of the *outcome* or the *process* of competency achievement. Educationalists indicate that this ought to be made explicit since having process and outcome mixed can be confusing for students and lecturers alike, and may affect grading. However, our experience with the contracts suggests that both are going on and are apparent in the

Figure 5.1 Extracts from two learning contracts

Objectives to include competencies	Resources and strategies	Evidence of achievement and reflection	Validation
Student 'V' 2.8.1 Critically examines the rationale for existing plans of care of clients with whom she is involved and becomes familiar with the associated theory and research.	Literature from files in office. Learning sessions with mentor. Reading past medical notes. Reading care plans associated with patient.	Being placed on a vascular ward made me explore more anatomy in books and literature because my knowledge was slim. Understanding it was important for me to become aware of many types of surgery carried out on the ward and the reasons behind it. Regarding a particular patient, I was totally unaware of the problems associated with diabetes. He had both of his legs amputated below the knee to aid his circulation. My research into diabetes showed me how the arteries and veins became narrower and how the blood circulation is limited. An ethical decision was made to remove his legs to help with this, and in a sense improve his quality of life. His care was specialized but not immediate. He was to rest and become used to his altered body image and achieve a better healthier life. He wasn't an elderly man and had very few family. I was surprised to see his health deteriorate so quickly. I had made a reasonable communication with him and found it a great shock when he suddenly died while I was not working. I had believed he would do well as to me he had made a reasonable recovery whilst I worked with him. It was only afterwards that I was told that sometimes this happens and deterioration is rapid. This was the first person I had cared for who had died. I felt disappointed and concerned. I wonder, if he was going to die soon, why he went through trauma, when even after his surgery he would be restricted considerably until he died.	We obviously needed to discuss this problem further as V didn't understand the reason for the surgery which was in fact palliative as the man wasn't expected to live many months. Without the operation he would have had intractable pain. Maybe being new to that ward scene there were so many facets to this problem all she managed to do was focus on the diabetes. She certainly developed a rapport with him but needed to be able to distance herself and see all the problems.

| Student 'R' 2.1.3 Identifies issues of a moral nature and justifies why they are considered to be so. Explore issues in the nurse–patient relationship. | Communication with mentor. Use of reflective diary. Literature on nursing ethics. | Nursed a seventy-six-year old man with leukaemia. He had had a recent splenectomy and his Hb was low. There was a possibility of blood transfusion. The patient and family seemed very anxious and were also quite knowledgeable about his condition and were expecting a transfusion. On a ward round, ECG results were discussed quickly without reference to the patient and using a lot of medical jargon. The consultant explained to the patient that following the splenectomy the spleen stops destroying RBCs and the Hb level should stabilize and so he didn't feel a transfusion was necessary. The medical and nursing staff chose not to communicate that the ECG had shown changes and a transfusion would therefore be a risk on the grounds that the patient was already extremely anxious. Callahan (1985) (Ethical issues in professional life, OUP) identifies a similar case of nursing compliance with medical deception (withholding of information would be a more neutral term) as a moral issue. Research cited in her book questions the value for the patient of being protected in this way. I personally believe that the nurse–patient relationship needs to be an adult–adult relationship to be truly therapeutic. Any deviation from this (such as protecting the patient by withholding information) must be examined. In the case of the patient described next I chose to openly discuss with him the risk that his stump revision could cause difficulties with the wearing of a prosthesis. My mentor and I were clear that our patient was already anxious about this and that it would be therapeutic for these anxieties to be dealt with openly. | R identified ethical issues well, acknowledging the validity of each decision and its importance. She contributed well to discussions and analysis of each situation, and saw the need to consider all angles/aspects when making ethical decisions. I would like to suggest therefore that competencies 3.1.11 and 3.1.2 have also been achieved. |

contracts. It is almost inevitable that the process of achieving competency is more clearly evidenced in Years 1 and 2, but we anticipate that contracts graded in Year 3 and particularly Year 4 will show more evidence of outcomes. The course is still being developed and work in this area will need to continue.

A second area of concern has been the potential influence of mentors on the type of contract written. As mentors help students reflect on their clinical experience and talk with them about their contracts, a situation may develop where the student take all the cues given by the mentor and in effect writes the 'mentors contract', anticipating that this will be rewarded by a high grade. Nursing does have some history of 'coaching' students to pass examinations. However, this has not been found to be a major problem, which may be due to my proximity and availability as the lecturer practitioner. Since I am clinically based, and have management responsibility, I am aware of the current clinical issues. This means that particular clinical experiences are already known to me and if they appear within a student contract I am in a position to challenge or reinforce. Similarly, the relationship and knowledge I have of mentors can be used to discuss a mentor's influence.

These strategies are not available when students are placed with mentors on wards not managed by me. This has been another issue for lecturer practitioners. When the mentor's manager is his or her own ward sister, rather than the lecturer practitioner, then the historical situation of the clinical teacher, negotiating access to students with the ward sister, may reappear. In this situation, the lecturer practitioner has to be sure of the appropriateness of placing students in clinical areas where they have no authority, and if necessary they may decide not to accede to demands to place students outside their own clinical areas.

Two further issues that have to be tackled are the design of the contract which students have contributed to, and a refinement of the competencies. Students' concerns about the overuse of jargon in this context are also being looked at. The whole process does not stand still, and lecturer practitioners are key people in ensuring the momentum is maintained.

Organizational issues

The managment of time, the demands of student contact and the analysis of a day's work into component parts are additional aspects worthy of consideration.

Time management and delegation

A comment often made to lecturer practitioners is – 'It sounds a great job but aren't you putting two jobs into one and getting run into the ground?'. This is a fair comment as there are a number of functions a lecturer practitioner fulfils. I have found that the way to ensure that it remains within the capability of one person comes down to two things: the confidence to delegate appropriately and managing my own time effectively.

Delegation of appropriate work is necessary in all areas of the job. I have devolved clinical responsibilities to the primary nurses within the ward team. Effective primary nursing ensures each patient has a named nurse who is managing the case and liaising as appropriate. I may be approached for advice but day-to-day issues are handled by the primary nurse. Ward management responsibilities are delegated to F grade team leaders, who are experienced nurses, well able and indeed expected to take discreet areas of overall ward management responsibility. These include off duty, day-to-day unit cover, managing staffing levels, orientating newly appointed staff and initiating staff appraisals for D grades. The development of an individual's ability to take on these areas of work is part of my responsibility.

Many administrative responsibilities are delegated to a secretary. Funding for the position is jointly from the education department and nursing staff budgets. Secretarial support is invaluable in securing the smooth running of mentoring arrangements, mentor preparation courses, and prompt response to correspondence. This lends an air of control to the situation. Secretaries are also helpful in fielding calls thus allowing that vital breathing space to assess how to respond to a particular request for time. It can be easier to say no when a response is considered first.

Teaching responsibilities have been delegated in one sense to the mentors, but there are also ways of delegating specific teaching to other ward staff who perhaps have an interest in taking up more formal teaching commitments in the future. For example, it may be appropriate for science graduate nurses working clinically to become involved in the theoretical pathophysiology modules, either as seminar group leaders or to lecture on specific subjects within the module. Again it is making use of the resources available and being imaginative in their deployment.

This delegation of work is helpful in freeing up time, but there is still plenty to fill the day. Managing time is important in helping me to retain control. Ensuring annual leave is taken regularly is helpful. Being aware of when learning contract interviews and other marking are due in advance, means that my diary can be organized appropriately. Making decisions about which meetings to attend and getting those dates into the diary early is also important.

There is still, however, no control over the demands that individual students make during term time. Crises come unannounced. I also function as professional tutor to a small number of students. I remain the student's professional tutor throughout the course and am the constant feature for them with responsibility for monitoring their overall progress. Inevitably some students use their professional tutor more than others, but accessibility and availability are important for all of them. Dilemmas do arise when I am faced with choosing between patient care and student time. In general patient care comes first, and as students become more familiar themselves with the uncertainty of practice their understanding of this dilemma improves. Nevertheless, the student will at times take precedence, and I have to be able to accommodate this, maybe missing a sisters' meeting or resource management meeting.

An integrated role

I have found that trying to analyse a day's work into its component parts is increasingly a false activity. It is more of an integrated role and sometimes two or more parts of the role are happening simultaneously. For example, discussing with a primary nurse a clinical issue she has asked advice on, may be part of a staff development role; with the student present it may encompass some mentor development responsibilities, looking at reflective skills; and it may raise a clinical issue that needs further review thus encompassing developing clinical practice. Dividing out that conversation and the ensuing work into its component part is a nonsense. The role is integrated.

Nonetheless, the reality is that student contact time is deemed an important indicator of educational involvement, whether through formal teaching, such as seminars, or individual time such as learning contract interviews. The time therefore has to be recorded. It is possible to divide the day into broad headings but there is a danger of losing the value of the integrated role which is in essence greater than the sum of the parts.

Clinical work

Managing the clinical part of the role is the icing on the cake. The personal satisfaction of being able to practise nursing relatively freely at a senior level is an added bonus. The benefits of practising in my own unit are that I am able to demonstrate for junior nurses the approach to nursing I would wish them to develop. As a consequence of dealing with problems I have become credible to the ward staff and they will come to me for advice with their own clinical problems. Credibility is also gained with other disciplines, particularly the doctors. Visible leadership is necessary to help other disciplines integrate with nursing, and senior medical staff are strongly supportive of the ward sister's function in this respect. Communication has been facilitated with medical staff as they have seen good clinical practice carried out by the senior nurse.

Most clinical time is functioning as an associate nurse. To take the primary nurse role is more demanding on time and may, if the patient's progress is pitted with troughs rather then peaks, mean excessive personal demands. Generally speaking, taking a primary nurse role is easier during vacation time than term time. Being an associate nurse has its advantages. Giving feedback to primary nurses on their care planning is more effective when I have been able to work with their patients. Likewise, assessing the standard of care is more possible when functioning as an associate nurse.

Areas for further work

As is always the way, the more one learns about a new approach, the more areas one can identify for further work. This is certainly the case with the role of the lecturer practitioner. There are three issues which appear to need more attention. First, the consistency of mentoring activity needs to be assured and more work should be done on the grading of practice. Second, the undergraduate course is still evolving and planning activities, especially in relation to the practice modules, remain high. To some extent they distort the real picture of workload in the longer term. This is an important consideration in the light of criticisms that the job is only achievable with immense commitment. Third, it seems likely that lecturer practitioners are here to stay. My personal experience suggests that the role is seen as desirable for aspiring nurse practitioners wishing to take on formal teaching responsibilities but not at the expense of leaving practice. It is therefore necessary to be explicit and develop appropriate career pathways culminating in lecturer practitioner posts, and to offer preparation for the role. Current post holders have a responsibility to contribute to this.

Conclusion

Working with students as a lecturer practitioner is both challenging and demanding. However, it offers a unique opportunity to influence the development of future nurses while still remaining skilled in practice. If well managed there is no doubt that the role can work, and is an effective way of bringing together the responsibility for managing patient care and for teaching students. Both groups learn from each other; students raise issues in practice which need review; mentors and lecturer practitioners guide and explore with students areas previously unconsidered, they provide students with strong role models and clarify their career aspirations.

This work is inevitably dynamic in nature – as a lecturer practitioner you cannot survive if working in a changing environment feels uncomfortable. The impact of integrated nursing education and practice demands continued development, and the trying out of new ideas and approaches. Over time these initiatives are increasingly shared among the nursing and health care team, but the learner's contribution is significant. This requires energy and enthusiasm, and for many in the NHS there are other significant demands on time and thinking. It may well be for this reason, plus the stresses of managing change, that this might not be a job that can be sustained for life!

References

Benner, P. (1984) *From Novice to Expert: Excellence and Power in Clinical Nursing Practice.* Addison-Wesley, California

Daloz, L. A. (1986) *Effective Teaching and Mentoring.* Jossey-Bass, San Francisco

England National Board (1987) *Institutional and Course Approval/ Reapproval Process. Information required, criteria and guidelines.* Circular 1987/28/MAT, ENB London

Fardell, J. (1988) The supernumerary student. *Nursing Times*, **84**(32), 32–33

Foy, H. and Waltho, B. J. (1989) The mentor system: are learner nurses benefiting? *Senior Nurse*, **9**(5), 24–25

Kershaw, B. (1990) Project 2000 – what do trained staff need for its successful implementation and development? *Senior Nurse*, **10**(1), 4–6

Morle, K. M. F. (1990) Mentorship – is it a case of the emperor's new clothes or a rose by any other name? *Nurse Education Today*, **10**, 66–69

Ogier, M. (1989) Breaking through the Darleck syndrome. *Nurse Education Today*, **9**, 341–346

6

The collegiate lecturer practitioner role

Ingrid Stevens*

Introduction

This chapter focuses upon a particular variant of the lecturer practitioner role which has become known as the 'collegiate model'. It elaborates how the job of one such 'collegiate' lecturer practitioner was established, and identifies the concepts and issues that are raised in light of the post holder's experience. It concentrates in the main on the initial stage of the job, and the development of the relationship with a senior colleague. However, the implications of subsequent changes, such as in the key personnel involved and within the job itself, are also touched upon.

The lecturer practitioner has been described by FitzGerald (1989) as a 'senior nurse who has mastery of practice, education, management, and research. Through demonstrating these collective skills she is able to lead a team of nurses delivering a professional service to patients, at the same time as developing personal skills and knowledge in her/himself and the nurses working alongside'. However, this combination of skills and areas of responsibility has been achieved in different ways and the actual job of the lecturer practitioner can vary widely. Typically, the lecturer practitioner takes on the role of a senior sister or a ward sister/charge nurse, and sometimes both roles, such as the authors of Chapters 4 and 5. However, in some service areas they may not

* This chapter has been written in collaboration with Judith Lathlean who studied this 'collegiate lecturer practitioner' throughout her first three years in post.

have sole managerial responsibility but be in collegiate relationship with one or more senior nurses or sisters, either in a ward, a group of wards – the unit – or a department. The precise nature of this relationship varies according to the particular circumstances and people involved, but in the instance described here, collegiality implies an equal partnership which achieves the collective skills required, and where the partners are cooperating towards the attainment of common aims.

Background to the post

Prior to the development of lecturer practitioners in the health authority, I was a clinical teacher supporting student nurses on the oncology ward where I subsequently became the lecturer practitioner. My clinical and teaching interests and experience were in oncology nursing, and as a clinical teacher I had a belief in the development of a clinical career structure which facilitates expert professional nurses to deliver patient care. This remains a commitment for me as a lecturer practitioner.

This post was planned jointly by me, the Senior Nurse for the oncology unit, the Director of Nursing Services for the hospital and the Head of the Polytechnic Department responsible for the undergraduate programme. It was agreed that the post would be funded 50% by the National Health Service (NHS) and 50% by the Polytechnic, though the Imperial Cancer Research Fund (ICRF), which has beds within the unit, agreed to pay half of the service contribution for a trial period of two years. The post was intended to be for the whole unit and included clinical practice development, management, education, support and research, in relation to NHS and ICRF nursing staff, and students in the undergraduate programme.

On taking up the post of lecturer practitioner, in the initial phase of the job I focused upon the ward that I was familiar with – a regional, adult, oncology ward, treating people admitted in the main with a variety of solid tumours by chemotherapy and radiotherapy. At this stage the ward had no sister and the Senior Nurse for the unit incorporated aspects of the sister role into his work. He was also responsible for the nurses and nursing practice in a sixteen-bedded hostel ward, an oncology out-patients department, and the X-ray and CT-scanning departments. This responsibility was subsequently extended to include the commissioning and establishment of the nursing service within a new pain relief unit, and an ICRF oncology research unit.

Evolution, boundaries and partnership

Transition from clinical teacher to lecturer practitioner

In the early days of the lecturer practitioner job, I was asked by the Senior Nurse, who was new in post, to interview for ward staff jointly with him. We developed the level of peer support that I had managed to achieve with other senior nurses and sisters I had worked with in the past as a clinical teacher. Further, the Senior Nurse requested that I spend more time in the ward, which would have suited my preference, that is, to teach only in my own speciality. His main concern, however, was to promote education and support for nursing staff as well as students. This equated with my belief that students' learning cannot and should not be separated from the development of clinical practice.

As a clinical teacher I had difficulty focusing only on student needs. There had always seemed to me to be an artificial boundary between learning situations and practice, and an inappropriate division of labour between those responsible for clinical practice and those attempting to facilitate student learning. The effective education of students, and the facilitation of their development into professional, competent nurses appeared to depend upon students actually experiencing good approaches to nursing care and high standards of practice. As a clinical teacher I could only offer suggestions regarding practice, and had no recognized time or responsibility for involvement in clinical practice planning and developments. As a lecturer practitioner I had both the time and the authority for these activities.

The process of evolution

When the nature of lecturer practitioner roles was debated in relation to the proposed nursing degree, and a number of different models were being promoted, a key principle behind all of them was the acceptance that the actual role of each lecturer practitioner should emerge from the local needs of the clinical area. It was clear, however, that the post would not be successful unless it was acceptable in the clinical area. In this respect, the time appeared to be right in the oncology unit, as demonstrated in the attitudes already described.

Although a job description was written at the start (Figure 6.1), the approach taken was experimental and open to negotiation and change, both through informal means and formally through an annual review process. Clinical, managerial, and educational functions were stated, and then related to aims which were identified by peer review. The aims in relation to research, however, were less clearly defined at the outset, but experience and role evolution have resulted in a clearer understanding of the research component over time. There has been an annual performance review, and the job description has been subject to modification in the light of experience.

Figure 6.1 Job description for a lecturer practitioner in a collegiate role

Job title   *Lecturer practitioner in an oncology unit*

Accountability to: • Senior Nurse (reciprocal, in relation to clinical and managerial work)
                     • Director of Nursing Services (in relation to clinical and managerial work)
                     • Head of the Polytechnic Department (in relation to undergraduate student responsibilities)

Responsibilities   The responsibilities will need to be clarified as the post evolves, but the following are the main areas that the post is likely to cover. The functions marked * overlap with those of the Senior Nurse, and their exact nature will need to be reviewed frequently.

Clinical function
   1. Practice as a primary nurse or associate nurse on a regular basis
* 2. Make explicit the nursing team's philosophy, identifying the most appropriate framework for practice, and ensuring that all staff understand the implications for practice

  ★ 3. Monitor and develop the quality and nature of
         nursing care and give regular feedback to the
         nursing team and Senior Nurse
  ★ 4. Demonstrate and develop research-based practice
         in the unit
  ★ 5. Ensure that the district policies are understood
         and adhered to in the unit
     6. Act as a nursing specialist, advising the ward and
         the unit

Educational function
  ★ 1. Develop and maintain the learning environment
         criteria for nursing students
     2. Identify and create innovative educational
         strategies for future nursing students
     3. Plan the programmes for all learners who visit the
         unit, and ensure that their mentors have a sound
         grasp of what is expected of them
  ★ 4. Assist all members of nursing staff to plan their
         personal development and education, and support
         them in developing a self-directed approach to
         learning
     5. Introduce and develop reflective practice
         appropriate for oncology nurses
  ★ 6. Promote personal and professional growth of the
         nursing team, implementing an appropriate
         performance review programme with the Senior
         Nurse
     7. Maintain own personal and professional growth
     8. Develop the ward learning resources
     9. Spend a minimum of two study days a month in
         reading and preparing for different aspects of the
         lecturer practitioner role
    10. Develop and clarify the lecturer practitioner role
         and share this information locally and nationally
    11. Act as a professional tutor for a small number of
         students

Managerial function
  ★ 1. Participate in recruitment, selection and retention
         of nursing staff, aiming to develop the most
         appropriate skill-mix
  ★ 2. Initiate and participate in ward and unit meetings
  ★ 3. Represent the professional and educational

interests of the unit at appropriate meetings and committees

★ 4. Understand the ward budget and its implications for education and development

★ 5. Cross-cover for Senior Nurse while on annual leave

★ 6. Support Senior Nurse and ward staff

Planning and negotiation

In the very beginning it was obvious that joint planning between the Senior Nurse and the lecturer practitioner was essential. Though this was to some extent a continuous process, certain phases of transition were found to occur, and three-monthly peer review and planning between the two of us was important. In this we needed to:

- Ensure a mutual understanding of our own personal and shared aims, and those for the unit;
- Agree on short- and long-term goal setting both for ourselves and for the unit;
- Identify areas of overlap between our roles and any potential conflict; and
- Offer each other peer support.

In this way trust continued to develop, and planned negotiation was found to be supportive and exciting. Rather than conflict arising, we pre-empted difficult situations by addressing problematic aspects together, and in doing so carried the burden together. Discussion helped us to clarify the issues and explore other points of view. In turn it helped to prevent professional isolation; the Senior Nurse had experienced this in previous posts, and expressed appreciation at being able to share problems with a senior colleague. A joint review of roles and the achievements in relation to our personal, combined and unit goals was mutually beneficial and helpful. We ensured that each of us facilitated the other's development. This was done in a number of ways, for example by:

- Sharing expertise – I helped the Senior Nurse review the gate theory of pain in relation to the pain assessment chart we were using. He in turn helped me to learn budgeting skills.

- Pooling expertise – neither of us had implemented team nursing, a model of nursing of patient participation in quite this way before. Discussion, peer support, and the resulting confidence gained, was felt by both of us to have promoted successful change.
- Covering each other's off-duty – this permitted one of us to attend study sessions or study days whilst the other was available in a unit managerial capacity.

It could be argued that the use of two senior nurses in this way is an expensive luxury. However, it could also be said that poor decision-making is costly. In an era of increased responsibility and pressures, for example, in relation to resource management, greater efficiency and effectiveness and quality assurance, the senior nurse role is undergoing rapid change. Those in post do not necessarily have all the requisite skills and expertise; these need to be gained, and certainly there is need for collegiate support.

Another important issue was the establishment of authority within the lecturer practitioner role. We followed the principle of gradually achieving authority through developing credibility within role, rather than through the power gained by being in a particular hierachical position. My managerial authority was reinforced when the Senior Nurse was absent and I was seen to make decisions and policy changes. The decisions and actions were then discussed upon his return. This was regarded as advantageous by both of us, since situations had been promptly dealt with, rather than being allowed, to use the Senior Nurse's description, 'to fester until [he] got back'.

Boundaries and partnership

The establishment of flexible role boundaries and an effective partnership were key issues in the development of a collegiate relationship between the Senior Nurse and myself. This was achieved by a process of continuous negotiation between us, to which our respect for each other's professional integrity and our shared understanding of the reciprocal accountability was critical. We were accountable to each other for our actions. We were also accountable to the nursing team, patients, and the Director of Nursing Services. In addition I was accountable to the Head of the Polytechnic Department.

Flexibility was facilited by us both recognizing the risks we were taking and the challenges we were facing, and by our acceptance that our roles were uncertain and liable to change. Importantly, it was essential for us to have clear overall aims to which we were both committed. These included:

- Maintaining and developing high standards of patient care, including achieving continuity of nursing care and developing research-based practice.
- Establishing a consistent approach to individual staff development and appraisal.
- Creating and maintaining an effective clinical learning environment for all staff.
- Setting up of staff support systems.
- Ensuring effective ward communication channels.
- Achieving the best use of the unit budget, in terms of both cost-effectiveness and benefits.

We thought of the achievement of these aims as a number of 'projects', and decided to identify which project each of us would lead. In relation to the aims we had three-monthly goals, to identify what we hoped to achieve and in which order. One example was the introduction of team nursing. We agreed that the Senior Nurse should lead this project, but I helped plan it as well as review achievements and difficulties. We supported each other and the nursing team throughout the changes. During this time I then planned the next phase of development. The nursing team unanimously disliked the assessment and care plan documentation. I prepared proposals to tackle this problem, and these included not only the documentation, but also the whole approach to patient assessment and care planning. The proposals, which were designed to dovetail with and reinforce the team nursing, were discussed with the Senior Nurse frequently. Consequently, as soon as the teams were ready, as a second 'phase' we were in a position to experiment with an alternative method of patient assessment and care planning. Since appropriate timing is a key factor when introducing change, we had to wait until the nursing team were ready to tackle 'phase two'. This proved to be six weeks later. During this time I introduced a staff support group as well, as it became evident that one was needed. Again, timing appeared to be a factor influencing the success of the innovation. The nurses had previously refused an offer to start a group, and it was only when this point had been reached that they were enthusiatic.

Another aspect influencing the boundary between our roles, and the nature of our partnership, was our joint 'skill mix'. We each identified and discussed our experience, special interests, expertise, and professional development needs. We were keen to use our unique combination of skills effectively and also to reflect on how we could individually develop our own roles. In this way we clarified and set our personal and combined goals, and coordinated the focus and timing of our endeavours.

The Senior Nurse had no direct involvement with the polytechnic department, but the establishment and evolution of the lecturer practitioner role within this department occurred simultaneously. As such I became heavily involved in numerous activities such as module planning and implementation and was required to attend many meetings concerned with the plannning and evaluation of the degree programme. I also retained some previous commitment to activities related to the traditional RGN course that was gradually being phased out during my first year in post. Inevitably workload commitments and departmental dead-lines clashed at times, and priorities had to be identified. Throughout this time peer support from the Senior Nurse was offered, accepted and valued.

Identifying and balancing workload commitments

Leaving aside the collegiate nature of the role, it has been important for the job to gain an identity of its own, and in working towards this end, a vital consideration has been the identification and balancing of all the different commitments. In the early days, goal setting, planning and prioritizing were not sufficient to enable me to meet all of my workload demands continuously and consistently. Having tried five different methods of organizing workload, I concluded that planning phases of activity was the most effective way forward. The phases have varied both in their nature and their determinants. So, for example, ward projects have given rise to some phases whereas, when the students come to the wards, the terms for the undergraduate programme have determined others.

With the best will in the world, and however good the planning, difficulties do occur owing to the unexpected. Each week I purposely tried to leave some unspecified time in my diary to accommodate the additional demands, such as a crisis with a personal tutee, or a ward issue which needed a prompt response. But inevitably this was not always possible with an already time-consuming job, or the extra demands were too substantial. As a result, I have learnt to maintain several simultaneous, long-term projects which can be picked up and restarted when 'flexitime' is available. And when I have been unable to achieve my weekly goals, low priority admininstration and meetings have just had to wait.

Thus good organization is clearly important. In addition, there are other key influences in the achievement of goals and the management of the workload, such as being realistic about goals, delegating some aspects of the work to others and gaining secretarial assistance. As already mentioned, setting goals for an entire ward or unit team needs to be flexible to accommodate team members' needs, and I found that it was important to ensure that staff were fully involved in and committed to our aims.

The ability to delegate is obviously dependent on the resources that are available, and in particular on the skills of those in potentially supportive roles. In our situation, we were helping team leaders to develop the skills required for such a senior clinical position. None of us knew the limits of the role, nor of the team leaders themselves. I have found it vital, in order to function fully as a lecturer practitioner, to be clear about the jobs of those in support positions, and to have the time to develop both people and roles.

The original plans for the lecturer practitioner role suggested that an important facet of making the job workable was the use of secretarial assistance. I have certainly found this to be a very helpful aspect, as was the availability of certain physical resources such as a reasonable photocopying budget. An inability to produce letters and teaching materials of an acceptable quality can be 'the final straw', when trying to develop a stressful, and at times uncertain, new role. In anticipation of such difficulties, the Senior Nurse and I converted a part-time auxiliary salary into secretarial funding. In addition, it has been possible to use some ward donations to pay for photocopying and activities arising out of development work, such as the printing of new care plans. I did this by establishing a specific nurse education ward fund, and donors have the choice of putting their money into one of three different funds.

One important facet of the job is that of working clinically on the ward. However, despite my intentions in this respect, I have found that regular and meaningful clinical practice as an associate nurse, providing continuity of care, has been difficult or impossible to achieve at times, owing to the numerous other activities already described. The way around this appears to be to plan periods of time – such as a few shifts or a week – in practice on the ward during the students' holidays. Even so, it is difficult to spend as much time as I would like working clinically. Despite this, I am confident that there will be more time when the under-graduate programme has run through once, when the module planning is complete and when our fundamental clinical practice development targets have been achieved.

Notwithstanding the lack of time for working with patients, I was able to 'keep in touch' with the ward. Since my office is very close to it, I visited most days. This has fostered regular communication with the staff, awareness of their ward situation and morale, and the sharing of advice information and ideas. The Senior Nurse attemped to function in a similar way, yet found the same as me – that it became increasingly problematic to provide regular nursing care and to give sufficient time to the ward.

Combining the lecturer practitioner and senior nurse role

Following the resignation of this particular Senior Nurse, there was a five-month gap before his successor commenced. During this time I attempted to undertake the combined job of senior nurse/lecturer practitioner. This was a tiring though enlightening experience. My conclusions were that with such a large, expanding unit, I could not fulfil all the aims of a combined post, especially since it incorporated the functions of a ward sister as well. The team leaders were stretched beyond their roles and skills by the level of delegation required. We identified the feasible boundaries of the team leaders' roles, and subsequently reviewed the ward nursing structure. Our commitment to the team nursing system remained, and the need for a ward sister became clear.

In those five months, priorities were achieved, but further development in the ward and unit was not possible. Major changes were taking place in the hospital that affected my responsibilities, such as the commissioning and combination of two units into one, the need to devise service contracts for the first time, and the presence in the unit of our first undergraduate students. These factors clearly had an effect on me and produced added pressures, but whether we would have achieved more than our priorities under different circumstances is open to conjecture.

Subsequent development and relationships

Following this early period in my job, two major changes in personnel have inevitably impacted on my role, the first being the appointment of a ward sister for the ward and the second, a new senior nurse for the unit with different skills, expertise and expectations. With respect to the ward sister, I have retained many of my clinical, management and developmental functions, though some of these are now shared, and the focus of my clinical support work has tended to shift to other parts of the unit. Furthermore, I am no longer involved in providing cover for the ward, nor in the traditional management activities that appropriately are undertaken by the sister, such as recruitment and the day-to-day support of her staff. Indeed the orientation of the job is now more overtly to the unit than to any particular part of it.

The nature of my role and relationship with the second Senior Nurse is rather different, in that she has a different kind of background, interests and expertise from her predecessor, and thus the division of responsibilities has inevitably altered. However, the processes that we have gone through to establish an effective way of working as senior colleagues is very similar, such as reviewing our strengths and inclinations, negotiating our mutual roles, and engaging in joint planning and evaluation.

Additionally, my role has been affected by my involvement as a student in a part-time Master's degree course in Advanced Clinical Practice (Cancer Nursing), both in terms of the time that I have needed to devote to the course and the increased knowledge and understanding gained in the clinical area. The experience has also convinced me that a master's level of education is necessary, to enable both the lecturer practitioner role and the post-holder to flourish, yet it is difficult to combine a very full job and concurrently undertake a demanding course of study, however beneficial it proves to be.

Conclusion

A fundamental aim of lecturer practitioners is to achieve a role which is a unified whole – delivering a professional service, leading a team and facilitating personal, team and nursing development. Historically there have been definite boundaries struck between clinical, educational, managerial, and research functions, but these are false divisions which are unhelpful in a number of respects, especially in the provision of good clinical care and in the education and development of students and trained staff.

In some of the models of lecturer practitioner, there has been an attempt to combine several aspects of these functions into the job of one person. My experience of collegiate roles raises the question of whether the nature of the speciality and such factors as the size of the unit influence the nature of the lecturer practitioner role. There is no definitive answer at present, but I believe that they have some bearing, and that it is appropriate for the roles to continue to differ, albeit within certain key principles as outlined in FitzGerald's (1989) description. Thus, in the unit where I work, I advocate a partnership between the jobs of senior nurse and lecturer practitioner. It could be argued that the success of such a partnership is heavily dependent on the people involved, and could therefore be problematic. However, having experienced two such collegiate relationships I am convinced that the benefits far outweigh the potential hazards. Importantly though, the principles and main aims should be jointly agreed, and the shared and individual accountability defined. Critically, an effective partnership is reliant on skilful negotiation between the parties.

On the positive side, partnership facilitates support, personal development, decision-making based on discussion, forward planning and review at a senior level. This sets examples for the rest of the nursing team, identifying the value of these activities and demonstrating the processes involved.

Redfern and Norman (1990) advocate the value of leadership in nursing, rather than a concentration on management alone. They identify characteristics of leaders which promote high quality. These include acting as a facilitator and risk-taker, and creating an innovative ward culture with confidence to enable nurses to use their creativity and leadership skills. These characteristics appear to be consistent with the aims and approaches identified above by the senior nurse and lecturer practitioner. There is still some way to go, but I believe that the development of the lecturer practitioner collegiate role has facilitated leadership in partnership.

References

FitzGerald, M. (1989) Lecturer Practitioner: Action Researcher. Unpublished MN Thesis, University of Wales

Redfern, S. J. and Norman, I. J. (1990) Measuring the quality of nursing care: a consideration of different approaches. *Journal of Advanced Nursing*, 15, 1260–1271

Part Three
The Australian experience

Helen Cox, Barbara Hanna and Kerry Peart

There is acceptance within the profession that nursing academics are generally well-grounded in the theoretical foundations of the discipline of nursing but are often less expert in clinical practice. They may have been superb clinicians at an earlier point in their careers, but as teachers they seldom practice in order to retain that expertise. Conversely, clinicians are usually experts in nursing practice, and are highly skilled in managing the complexities of their practice worlds, but have often been less well-grounded in the theoretical foundations of the discipline. Nursing is essentially a practice discipline. Nursing, however, is taught by people who are in the main, removed from practice. How then is it possible for academic nurses to produce the continuing supply of new members of the workforce who will be able to function in the real world of nursing? This is a question that has been the focus of argument and debate for years. The assumption is that a gap exists between theory and practice or between service and education; that each is mutually exclusive, and that strategies are needed to bridge that gap, uniting the two worlds. Presumably this means having academics somehow involved in practice and to have clinicians somehow more involved in the theoretical development of nursing.

Questions are raised about whether practitioners really do practice without using theory, or without theorizing, and whether academics realistically conceptualize and theorize practice without practising (Pearson, 1988). Indeed, are theory and practice separate, or do they really interpenetrate each other, as Smyth (1987) argues, with elements of each existing in the other?

There is debate about whether this theory–practice gap really does exist, and if it does, whether it is unhealthy. However, the need for professional nurses to inhabit each world is real, whether it is perceived as bridging the gap or whether it is recognition of the fact that theory can be derived from practice just as importantly as practice can derive from theory. Each world presents an important place to explore for people who normally inhabit the other.

It is with Smyth's arguments in mind and with the aim of exploring ways of 'knowing nursing', that the Faculty of Nursing in this particular Australian university has pursued models which interweave academic and clinical roles for staff. The purpose of this part of the book is to present the three models in use, with clear descriptions of why and how they were implemented, and outlining the benefits and difficulties encountered in each.

The three models in use are:

- The *Lecturer or Tutor/Clinician Role*, where all full-time members of the academic staff are expected to spend 20% of their year engaging in faculty practice, that is in clinical work.
- The *Clinician/Lecturer Role*, where full-time expert clinicians are seconded from their clinical agency to the faculty for 20–60% of their time to engage in teaching.
- The *Joint Appointment Role* where two nurses are employed each with 50% of their time as an academic, and the other 50% of their time as a charge nurse in a Professional Clinical Nursing Research Unit.

Although the area of emphasis is different with each role, all of them are designed to offer both professional and academic leadership to students. In addition, each role is designed so that the incumbent is able to pursue and research nursing intellectually, and to make significant contributions to both of the areas in which he or she is involved.

The following three chapters describe these models of practice which have successfully blended the worlds of education and service: the implementation of faculty practice for academic staff; the employment of clinician/lecturers as members of faculty; and the exploration of the possibilities in joint appointments. In each of these roles the ultimate aim is the same; to examine and improve our own practice and that of our students. Each role promotes the centrality of practice to nursing, and each offers a rich and unique opportunity to explore the ways in which theory drives practice, and the ways in which practice generates theory.

Each role requires a blend of different and similar skills. The academic in faculty practice is not purporting to be a clinical expert, the clinician/lecturer is not purporting to be a skilled academic, though these roles will result in increasing skill development. The joint appointee shares an equal requirement for skill in both areas.

Each role offers different insights into nursing. The academic in faculty practice has the opportunity to explore nursing from a myriad of perspectives, and is perhaps the most privileged of all roles since the person undertaking this practice is not on staff, nor in a position of responsibility in the agency and is therefore somewhat protected. If time can be allocated, the opportunity for reflection on, and in practice is rich and full of promise. The clinician/lecturers are protected to a degree in their university role, since they are not chairing units but work under the direction and supervision of a member of the academic staff. Their clinical role in their own agency is usually in a senior position, and they have the opportunity to reflect on that role in a way that is enhanced by their contact with the course, the academic staff and the students whose fresh perspectives on nursing are described. The joint appointee has no inbuilt protections – both people are in positions of responsibility in both agencies, being a charge nurse in one and unit chairperson in the other. The protections have to come from the administrative structures and processes in each agency, and from their colleagues. The joint appointment model may be the most problematic and yet the most potentially rewarding model of them all. The ways in which each aspect of this role reflects back to a greater understanding and appreciation of the richness of nursing are outlined.

The descriptions of each model contain notions of threat, challenge and commitment. But the notions are different for each person. For Helen in faculty practice, threat is about returning to practice and being observed as not confident and competent yet while holding a position as an academic, teaching about nursing, clearly shows a contradiction that would invoke criticism. For Barbara and Kerry it is about taking up an academic role, with no formal preparation for teaching. For Shirley and Pauline the threat comes from the expectation of being change agents. However, everyone operates out of some position of safety, having at least one foot in familiar territory.

For each person, challenges are accepted positively, but constraints are recognized and lamented; lack of time is a problem identified by each person, as is the physically and emotionally draining nature of the duality of roles. The need for keenly developed communication skills is another theme, and is isolated as a critical factor which determines the success or failure of the role.

It may be because of a sense of experimentation, or innovative leadership, or just the nature of the people attracted to this faculty and what it is trying to achieve, but whatever the origin, the clear sense of commitment must be recognized. It is commitment which turns something from being burdensome and problematic into a challenge, and it is a sense of excitement for what is happening in the 1990s in nursing which sustains the challenge.

References

Pearson, A. (1988) *Theorising Nursing: The Need for Multiple Horizons.*

National Nursing Education Conference, Expanding Horizons in Nursing Education Perth, Western Australia

Smyth, W. J. (1987) *A Rationale for Teachers' Critical Pedagogy: A Handbook*. Deakin University Press, Geelong

7

The lecturer clinician role: faculty practice

Helen Cox

Introduction

Written in to the terms of employment for full-time members of academic staff, no matter whether they are contracted or tenured, is the expectation that all will engage in faculty practice. In this particular context, the word 'faculty' refers to the teaching staff of a college or university rather than to a group of related subject departments within the university. Faculty practice recognizes the need for academic staff in a professional school to maintain a focus on clinical practice. The requirement is that each member of staff will spend 20% of his or her year working in a clinical setting, engaging in direct client care rather than being involved with student teaching and supervision.

There is no stipulation given regarding the location of anyone's faculty practice, and staff members may have entirely different reasons for choosing their particular area of interest. At present there are lecturers and tutors undertaking faculty practice in critical care units, in professorial clinical nursing development units, in elderly care areas, in mental health units, in community health, in midwifery and in various acute care areas. Some staff members wish to maintain skills in a particular clinical field, some are collecting data for research, others are exploring nursing and increasing their depth of questioning about the phenomena that they encounter in nursing, and the therapeutic nature of nursing itself.

Part of organizing faculty practice involves discussion with the Dean of the Faculty, (or Head of Department) regarding where one wishes to work and why. Negotiations are carried out between the Dean and the Director of the agency and formal contacts are negotiated. This is, in part, to arrange such matters as insurance cover and work care responsibilities, but it is also to ensure that both institutions are clear about the purpose of the faculty practice. A very important consideration in the eyes of the Australian Nursing Federation, is that we are not seen to be taking positions from registered nurses in this area; faculty practice positions are supernumerary, paid by the university, and cannot be used to replace agency staff on sick leave. If it fits with the aims of the placement, the staff member will arrange to take a client case load on the day by negotiating with the Charge Nurse, but will not take the work of a permanent member of the team.

The 20% replacement is flexible and can be done on one day per week; one week in five; one month in five or whatever arrangement suits other commitments both within and outside of the university.

The decision

I had been teaching in a hospital School of Nursing for some twelve years prior to joining the faculty at the university. The only clinical experience I had over that time was as a clinical teacher, and even then mostly with pre-registration students. I was always acutely aware that whilst working with students, I was only maintaining those skills that were relevant to the level of the student. In the later years I did no clinical teaching at all, so by the time I was thinking about faculty practice, I was sadly out of touch and feeling quite vulnerable. This was probably the main reason why it took me some time to decide where I wanted to practice, where I would be able to practice, and for what purpose I would practice, and then to arrange the necessary contract.

It is said, and it was certainly my fear, that the longer I spent away from clinical nursing practice, the greater would be the gap between what I talked about in the classroom and laboratories, and what I was actually able to do in the real world of nursing. On the very few occasions that I was involved in any direct care, apart from in my capacity as a teacher, I was left in no doubt at all that my confident, fluid and skilled practice had altered markedly.

Was it any wonder that the thought of returning to practice was so alarming!

The university has a practice driven curriculum, practice being espoused as the central focus of the faculty. Given that this university was where I wanted to be, faculty practice was to become a part of my life – and quickly.

My clinical background had been predominantly in the acute care field, with my first love being neurosurgery. Going almost anywhere other than acute care would be to break quite new ground for me, yet I felt that to practice in acute care was really out of the question. There would be far too many new things going on that I would have no knowledge of at all, and I was already so rusty on the old things, particularly the technology. I was embarking on faculty practice for me as a nurse, not for me as a teacher, so I made the intentional decision to be kind to myself (and to those for whom I would care!) and concentrate on my 'people skills'. I was particularly interested to see if I had retained any of those 'knacks' of practice which we develop over time. I knew that once I had a whole repertoire of these.

After much deliberation, I decided that my purpose in engaging in faculty practice would be to think about nursing, to reflect on what nursing means to me; how and why I do things that I do in the way that I do them; what beliefs I hold about nursing practice; and how they relate to the reading and studies that I continue to do in nursing. This meant that I would be constantly examining my own practice, rather than the practices of those around me, unless those practices challenged some belief that I held.

I had visited a sixty-bed private nursing home in the region, to organize student placements, and was impressed with their standards of care. I had spent some time caring for the elderly in the past, and considered it an important clinical area. I felt that this could be an area that would challenge me, the nurse, rather than me as technologist – just what I was looking for as my initial foray into faculty practice.

I approached the Director of Nursing of this agency with a request that I commence practice there. She appeared somewhat taken aback, but she agreed. The staff were supportive of me, once they overcame their suspicions. I had to prove that I could lift, that I could get my hands dirty like anyone else, and that I could work hard before they relaxed enough with me to begin to get to know me.

Although each night I could feel every bone and muscle in my body, I enjoyed my time there immensely. I have the utmost respect for nurses who have the stamina to do this day after day.

I worked at this particular agency over a period of one year, and then, feeling braver, I negotiated to move to a Professorial Clinical Nursing Unit at a nearby large acute hospital. My reasons for engaging in faculty practice at this agency remained the same as my initial purpose, but I felt I was ready to begin to pick up on some of the other skills that I once used so confidently.

I tried very hard to get to these agencies one day each week, but inevitably, the pressures of my multiple roles in the faculty led to missing many. The clause I put in the contracts about not being used to replace staff almost became redundant, as any attempt on their part to use me in this way would have failed miserably – I was not to be relied on. My arrangement sometimes had to be 'if I turn up, I am here!'. On those occasions I had to be sure to arrive early before a shift so that the days plans would not be put out if my arrival was unexpected.

Experiencing faculty practice

The tool that I chose to help me with my exploration of nursing was a personal professional journal. Journals are an effective means of assisting people to become more reflective as practitioners. I have kept a journal for some time now, adding entries for every clinical day in as much detail as possible. Sometimes I write about all of the things that I do, see or hear. I write about how they affect me and what images or thoughts they conjure up for me. Other times I write in detail about a specific situation that had an impact on me for some reason.

Over time, I return to my writing and read it again. I look for patterns and themes in my journals. I have found so many interesting things about me as a person and as a nurse, and I have found so many interesting things about nursing. For example, I have been dismayed to find that I am a nurse who 'does things' for people when for years I have espoused the belief that I encourage independence in people. There are many areas where I have found that what I have said I do, or believe in, is not matched at all by what I really do. I have been thinking deeply about this, trying to work out how aspects of my practice have evolved as they have, why I have held habits, rituals and espoused, but not used, theories dear for so long without knowing. Where I have surfaced anomalies I am faced with the question of just how I am going to go about altering my practice.

Re-reading the initial entries in my journal evokes the anguish I felt: the sleepless night before day one; the discovery that I had been 'set up' by a senior member of staff as an 'expert from the university' and that they were 'so lucky to have me'. I wrote about how I had to locate this member of staff and tell her what this was doing to my stress levels! I had hoped fervently to be low key and invisible on this first day, just so that I could at least find my way around and get some sense of the place.

Proof of this anxiety state was located in my writing about the second day, a week later. I was living some eighty kilometres from this agency, not yet having relocated, so it was about an hour's drive from home. I had arranged to begin at 7.00 a.m. and my long-suffering husband drove me there. At the age of forty I had just learned to drive, in order to apply for this position at the university, and I was still scared of driving. If I could get out of it, I did. After delivering me to the agency he went on to the coast to do some fishing, with the strict instruction to return for me at 12.30. I had decided that five and half hours would be enough. I rationalized that at the time, I had so much else to do! But it is clear to me from my journal that it was anxiety about whether I would cope and this was a sort of escape hatch. When he arrived at 12.30, I was really in the swing of things and was reluctant to leave. I felt that the morning had been fine and that I had made a reasonable contribution. From then on, my journal tells me that I settled in and didn't have this frantic urge to run away again.

Faculty practice days became ordinary. I did different things in each agency, but basically I washed people, or helped them to bath or shower; I helped them to dress, and sit out of bed; I took people for walks; I did dressings; sometimes I gave out medications; sometimes I monitored intravenous therapy, and I fed people. All the while, I chatted with people, for all the reasons that all nurses do. My day was mainly the same as most nurse's days within the areas that I chose to practice, but with the absence of any administrative role. It all seemed very ordinary, but my journal tells me that there is quite often nothing ordinary at all about the effect of what nurses do.

The journal as a teacher

I have already mentioned the dependence/independence theme that emerged from my journal. This began in a rather amusing (though only in hindsight) anecdote that I have related at many conferences and seminars on the subject of reflective practice. It involved working as a facilitator in a session with students where we were using professional actors as patients. We interrupted the long morning for a cup of tea, whereupon I proceeded to assist the actor, a fit and able young man, to remove his leg plaster and put on his trousers. It was only when I was crouching on the floor, holding his trousers for him to put his legs into, that I realized what I was doing.

Initially I wrote this up in my journal because I was so embarrassed, but also because it was a fine example of becoming hooked into the role. There had been so much criticism that using actors as patients was not realistic! The real lesson only revealed itself over time, as I explored my journal and found many occasions where, when on faculty practice, I performed tasks for people that they were quite capable of performing for themselves. My espoused theory – that I encouraged independence – was not in use at all. There was obviously some other theory that drove my practice of which I was completely unaware.

On later reflection, trying to unravel my history to make sense of this, I recognized a shadow from my past. After the death of my mother when I was quite small, I went to what I remember was called a 'foundling home'. I was cared for by mothercraft nurses, and developed a special fondness for one of them. She took me everywhere with her and, under her supervision, I fed, washed and dressed babies, played with them and helped to make up formulae. When I ran in fear of the belching sterilizers and bulk milk boilers she protected me. I loved every minute of it. I wanted to be like her. Clearly for me there was a direct link between 'nursing' and 'mothering', one that I had never recognized. My next task was to examine whether this definition of nursing was appropriate, and clearly it was not. I had to work on new ways of knowing nursing.

Now that I am aware of this anomaly, I can see clearly many examples in my practice where I was equating nursing with mothering. It is odd how transparent it is to me now yet it was so completely invisible before.

Another interesting lesson that I learned from reflecting on faculty practice occurred when I was caring for Betty, a woman with Down's Syndrome. In my journal I made the comment that I felt uncomfortable with people with intellectual disability, and on reflection have avoided them if I could. Now I ask myself, is it that my world can only tolerate physically impaired people, or is it that I fear what I don't understand? On this particular day I fed Betty, I was awkwardly trying to talk to her but getting no response. It was only when I gently touched her cheek that she quickly turned her face into my hand, opened her eyes and gave me a huge smile. We couldn't communicate with words really, but she did say a clear 'yes' to an occasional question. I worked hard at my relationship with her and found that I could turn around many of my beliefs and practices. This led to pondering the act of relating to patients broadly. I could look back through the years and locate examples of giving glib answers to confused people, humouring them or acting up for my workmates. I thought about this and studied my relationships with the people for whom I was caring now in faculty practice. In my journal I wrote:

> all of the ways I have related to patients before do not fit the me I am now, it will be interesting to explore this further because there are many confused people here. (Cox 1988)

An entry in my journal some weeks later read;

> I feel better about talking to residents now. I feel I have a balance of sensible talk and entering fantasies. I think I do both naturally and sensitively and I am very different now from years ago when I went along with fantasies but often laughed at the patient. I recall lots of times when I acted insensitively and I wonder now what was happening for me at the time; was I frightened? Was I rejecting something that I didn't understand? I feel so much of my past life was spent in some frozen state of suspension. I was so young when I was young! I wish that I had been more mature, there were so many

opportunities for learning that I missed by not being ready. (Cox 1988)

Thus there was much that I was able to learn about myself as a nurse and as a person in this valuable time. I also discovered how much I could pass on to the students. In the classroom I was able to draw on such up-to-date examples. For instance, I could say when talking about caring for someone who had experienced a cerebral vascular accident 'Those of you working at ★ ★ ★ Nursing Home will recall Mr Jones, and how he was last week. Yesterday when I was there I found that he had had a stroke. He is clearly distressed and is having quite some difficulty in communicating to staff. This is what we worked out together over the span of the day . . .' or 'Remember Mrs Jacobs? Since you last saw her she has had her leg amputated. The reason for that was . . . and we had to be very careful in planning her care for the day to . . .' – which meant that they had a clear picture of the some effects of the condition for the person, and they also had a picture of what they would find and need to work with on the following day when caring for these very people. It gave so much more credibility to the discussion than if I was dredging up some memory from the past, or making up some scenario. These people were alive and known to them. The students could arrive at the agency the next day having researched some aspect of the condition or the specific problem and with some ideas to share about what they might do about it that day.

Enjoying faculty practice

There have been many rewards to all of those days in faculty practice that I have managed so far. A major one is the discovery that my people skills have not left me. Indeed I believe that I am richer for maturity, for parenting, and for the thinking and reflection that has been a part of my teaching career in order to teach students about nursing in sensitive ways.

Over time I found that I developed an increasing sense of familiarity with the ward, its staff, its clients, its culture and mood. I found that the feeling of confidence kept increasing and I was able to relax about being there. Sometimes I left the ward knowing that my being there had made a difference, sometimes to clients, sometimes to staff.

I even found that my body started to learn to cope with the physical demands. As I had expected, immersing myself in the everyday world of patients kept me aware of the complexities of health care issues and of clinical practice. I was able to share with other staff in the solving of problems, developing of knowledge about nursing and researching of options in care. All of these reflected in my teaching and in the ways I was able to contribute to areas within the curriculum.

There was also a considerable advantage to be gained for both the clients and the students, in my becoming familiar with the culture, policies and protocols of the agency. I gained a greater understanding of each patient – their difficulties, their likes and dislikes in terms of care – than I would have had if I was there as a clinical teacher with students only. This, I am sure, served to reduce the gap that students experience when they move from the classroom to the clinical setting and experience 'reality shock'.

Mauksch (1980) points out that professionals in fields such as medicine, dentistry, architecture and the ministry teach through their practice. She asks how it has come about that so many teachers of nursing teach practice but do not engage in it themselves. My experience of engaging in both faculty practice and clinical teaching in the same agency altered my teaching significantly.

One particularly important facet of the experience has been the way in which I have been able to see my journal as a gold mine of raw data about nursing. The richness in those pages is amazing, and I find new things every time I read them. I have used material from my journal in writing several assignments for the course work component of a Master of Nursing Studies Course. One was a detailed account of my own practice, analysed for the theories that drive my practice. Another was an account of suffering, a case study completely derived from describing and analysing the experiences of one patient and those caring for him throughout an extremely agonizing time in his life. I have also used journalling as a component part of action research methodology, working with clinicians as we explore the nature of empathy. Together in our journals we are locating some rich and lovely truths about nurses and nursing.

I am convinced that journalling practice will, wherever possible, remain a major part of my continuing studies and research.

The problems of faculty practice

Although I was confident about the what and why of the clinical tasks that needed to be done, I had been quite worried about whether I would manage the how. The time spent in the first agency, however, revealed that I could remember how to do anything that was required of me. That was a relief, and it freed me to get on with what was really important in care. In the second agency it was not quite so easy. Why is it that I never could, and still cannot, thread intravenous tubing through sleeves, or catheter tubing through pyjama pants, without everything ending up back to front and in knots?

A really difficult problem was educating staff to see me as an ordinary person. I was initially seen as an 'ivory tower academic' who couldn't 'do' nursing, or who wished to observe but not get involved in the rather messy chaos of the real world of nursing practice. Conversely, I was seen as the all knowing, wise expert who has the solution for all problems. Staff in both clinical agencies had certain expectations about my level of knowledge and skill, and about what I could contribute to the agency and its practices in terms of change. There was also an expectation that I would conduct research as it is traditionally understood. My journalling and reflection for personal research into nursing was not quite what they expected and/or hoped for.

Time became somewhat of an enemy. There was no one to assist with my academic responsibilities whilst I was at the agency. That work just piled up and waited for me. The 'at home' work load was often quite high. In addition, writing in my journal at the end of a day that started at 7.00 a.m., finished at 3.00 p.m. only to resume again half an hour later at the university so that I didn't fall too far behind in my other roles, was another issue. Yet if I didn't write the same day, it was easy to slip into the trap of being too busy to write at all. Information not captured quickly was sometimes lost. This was a problem when research into my practice was my reason for being there.

There has been criticism levelled at the lack of continuity for clients when faculty members only work sporadically. In the first agency, the clients and staff came to know me quite well, I was with the same client group each week in my own practice, and again when I was supervising students. In addition, it must be remembered that this was a nursing home with a stable, relatively long-term population. The second area that I chose, the hospital setting, was different in that the patient population changed quickly, but the patients appeared to accept constant new faces amongst the staff. Often, in our large acute hospitals, casual staff are employed either from the hospital 'bank' or from employment agencies. If it was a problem in either agency I was not aware of it.

There was another probably minor, but interesting, dimension. Nursing was relatively new to the university, but the people in this region had fought hard to have it established. Most of the people under my care were genuinely interested in what we were doing and how we were faring, so a common feature of the day included enquiries from people who had championed the university so strongly, about what they could expect in return, in terms of quality of care, from our graduates. In one sense, as their teacher, my own skills and knowledge were under scrutiny. This was both a source of pleasure and a continuing source of tension.

By far the most criticism about faculty practice is directed to making it obligatory, and to its potential for overloading the willing workhorse. The charge is that it fosters burnout in staff who are expected to teach, to continue personal studies for higher degrees, to research, to publish, to be involved in professional organizations and activities, to be involved in committees and other activities both within the faculty and within the university broadly. My own experience is that this is true. A careful balance is essential, as is a recognition that sometimes you simply cannot manage it all this week, and that there is nothing wrong with that. Careful attention needs to be directed by the university and faculty administrators to structures and processes that support staff engaging in multiple roles.

An interesting model which has been put forward by Woodruff (1988), in an attempt to address this very issue, is for each member of staff to negotiate with the Dean or Head of Faculty for whatever the emphasis is to be for all or a portion of the coming year. In one year the emphasis may well be on clinical practice for whatever reason. In another year, however, the emphasis could be on writing and publication, so that the actual time devoted to faculty practice for that year or portion of the year may decrease. Woodruff suggests that adopting this sort of model would 'rescue us from the historic expectation that we must attempt to be all things to all people'. Each of the role components that a university lecturer has involves hard work, each deserves its own emphasis and development. Recognizing what component is due for particular attention and time devoted to it is an important skill in itself. In some ways I have had to adopt this model for myself, simply to survive.

According to Christman (1980), the full professional role of any nurse incorporates education, research, consultation and service. It is not good enough to plead 'no time' and therefore do nothing about taking on board the full range of responsibilities. Workable models must be investigated. While it is recognized that nursing in Australia is new to universities, part of carving out our niche in that world is to persevere with our development in all of these spheres. Thus, in addition to out teaching role, we must pursue higher degrees, keep up to date with clinical advances, pursue questions about nursing in research and communicate to the nursing profession and to the academic world what it is we are doing and discovering. We cannot afford to place all of our emphasis on teaching. No one denies that these are difficult and demanding expectations, but there is recognition that we have little option but to strive for such goals and indeed as a profession, we would wish to do so.

I do not wish this chapter to leave an impression that faculty practice is too difficult. I would like to leave the impression however, that it does require commitment, hard work, a valuing of the practice nature of nursing, and not to be forgotten, it requires stamina.

References

Christman, L. (1980) *An Organisational Perspective for Nursing Practice.* American Nurses Association Convention, Houston, Texas, 9–13 June

Cox, H. (1988–1991) *Personal Professional Journal.*

Mauksch, I. (1980) Faculty Practice: a professional imperative. *Nurse Educator*, May–June 1980, 21–24

Woodruff, A. (1988) *What is Faculty Practice?* Bridging the Gap Conference Proceedings, Deakin University, Geelong

8

Clinician lecturers in nursing

Barbara Hanna and Kerry Peart

Introduction

The Pre-Registration Course curriculum document cites the role of the clinician/lecturer in nursing as a role which . . . 'offers professional and academic leadership to students in the school of nursing, particularly in the area of clinical nursing practice' (Deakin University, 1988, p. 19). The purpose of the role is to provide the practice expertise in the integration between theory and practice. Clinician/lecturers are nurses who have achieved expert status in practice and whose task it is to merge what is taught in the classroom and what is practised in the clinical setting, whilst raising questions for students to explore further. The philosophy of the faculty supports this, arguing that:

1 Nursing is a practice discipline.
2 Clinical expertise can be achieved through sound theoretical preparation and thorough practical knowledge derived from the experience of practice.
3 Development of the discipline of nursing requires successful integration of theoretical thinking, empirical research and creative practice. Therefore change must incorporate both academic and clinical strategies (Deakin University, 1988, p.11).

Between 40 and 80% of a clinician/lecturer's time must be spent in a senior role in clinical practice while the remaining time is taken up with the preparation and conduct of learning experiences as a university lecturer in nursing. Variation exists in terms of employment, with some clinician/lecturers being full-time workers seconded from their agency, while others are part-time in agencies and employed separately by the university.

Clinician/lecturers are appointed with specific expertise and experience within a defined area of nursing. Their skills, while practical, should however be readily communicable to students. Thus a sensitivity towards the needs of students must also be apparent. A good working relationship between the university and health agency needs to be facilitated if students are to be well accepted, while ongoing communication is vital to iron out the problems that can, and do occur once students begin their placements. There is also a requirement that further study must be pursued, and an expectation that there will be some attendance at the regular staff development sessions conducted for all academic staff on the university campus.

The specific tasks of the clinician/lecturer may involve giving lectures and tutorials, and conducting nursing science laboratories and arts laboratories sessions. A necessary part is negotiating with nursing agencies and staff, and assisting students in gaining meaningful experiences out of their clinical placements and encouraging them to reflect on their experience in order to make sense out of them. Because the clinician/lecturer is essentially a clinical expert, clinical teaching and demonstrations in the nursing science laboratories make up the largest component of the role, although a valuable amount of formal lecturing and tutoring is built in.

Such a position offers the practising clinician the opportunity to become a part-time member of the university faculty with the status of a lecturer. This is both daunting and challenging for any practice-oriented nurse, game enough to take on such a task, for it involves serving two masters and attempting to meet the expectations of both. On one hand, health agencies often adhere to traditional philosophies, whereas tertiary programmes may espouse different ways of thinking. The clinician/lecturer is in a position to challenge the health care system, and create change which ultimately benefits not only the health care setting, but the university and the practitioner as well.

In the past many nurses who climbed the career ladder had nowhere to go clinically after they had achieved senior positions. The choices open to them were to go into management or to become nurse educators if they wanted to further their career goals. For those making such choices, movement away from clinical nursing was inevitable. This may be the ultimate goal for some nurses, but others whose clinical skills and expertise were recognized as excellent may be considered a sad loss to the field of direct patient care. The creation of clinician/lecturer posts is one way out of this dilemma.

When first notified of such an appointment, excitement at the prospect must be one of the initial emotions experienced. For those nurses who have always been interested in the 'education' aspect of nursing, it provides a great opportunity to 'try it out' without losing the valued practical skills of nursing acquired over many years. Closely behind comes fear that the appointed person may not feel educationally qualified to deal with university students who expect tertiary qualified lecturers. An example of this, in action, is the situation in which it would be virually impossible to expect clinician/lecturers to grade the students' work if they had no comprehension of what was a satisfactory standard of work for a university paper.

Getting started

Clinician/lecturers are appointed after meeting the selection criteria and undergoing comprehensive interviewing. They are initiated into the philosophy of the faculty through a series of meetings before commencing their new role, which has proved invaluable in coming to terms with current nursing thinking. Many nurses may never have heard of, or truly understood, the nursing process, primary nursing and much of the current language, let alone know what a nursing model is. These questions are answered over time and through further personal study, which is a requirement for all academic staff. In addition, staff undergo in-service training in classroom teaching. However, none of this prepares clinicians fully for some of the frustrations they inevitably encounter;

> I was notified two weeks before semester began that a position was available for a clinician with midwifery skills. I would be involved in coordinating a component of the undergraduate programme that specifically involved my clinical area and that would mean working

with students both in the hospital setting and the university. Because of the required hours of both the university and the hospital few people were capable of taking on both part-time positions simultaneously. I worked suitable shifts that would make it possible to fit both jobs into my life. When I was asked to accept the role of clinician/lecturer I promptly said yes. What a great opportunity I told myself. But the next day I remember thinking 'How am I going to organise three children, two jobs and one degree course into each week?' I started work for the university two weeks later with little idea of how or what I would teach students, and spent the first few weeks trying to placate my workmates who kept comparing this first group of university students with the much more practically skilled hospital trainees. The differences were so blatant that initially they believed we would return to the more 'superior' hospital trained nurse any day. The university, my colleagues believed, was just wasting its time. The mistakes of one student were deemed the fault of the whole system. I was viewed at times with distrust when I tried to make staff understand how new these students were to our hospital culture. (Peart, 1990)

The educational role

The central role of the clinician/lecturer is facilitating the acquisition of clinical skill in the laboratories at the university and in clinical agencies where students are placed. Teaching clinical skills is the 'bread and butter' of clinical nurse, after all, every nurse knows how to take a blood pressure reading or do a simple dressing. Teaching such basic procedures to students in a laboratory can be very different from practising on real people in hospitals and the integration of those two modes of teaching has been found to be helpful.

We had been through giving injections in science laboratories, going over correct site, method, protocols for having the drug checked and even drug calculations. The students were nervous but ready to give their first injection on a live human being. One particular student had anxiously practised over and over again on a piece of sponge before my arrival, knowing that I would be the one to take him through the procedure for the first time. The client was to be given a pre-medication by us before being taken to theatre. We followed the well learned protocol and arrived at the client's bedside, injection in hand. The student became catatonic, unable to move a muscle. I placed my hand over the student's and guided the needle in. With this move, he seemed to awaken and finished giving the injection himself. The client praised him for being so gentle which gave his confidence a great boost. Not knowing how students are going to react calls for quick thinking but so far they have not thrown anything at me that I haven't been able to deal with. (Peart, 1990)

The lessons taught in science laboratories are second nature to clinicians who have practised these skills until they are expert. Students, no matter how hard they practice in a laboratory, will always react differently when confronted with real life. Part of a clinican's role is to assist them through the transition from hypothetical to reality using the 'tricks' that they have mastered with time. Because the clinician is a 'real' member of staff in the clinical agency, as well as a university employee, they are familiar with the local rules and fluent in the norms of the agency. Hence, they are not 'foreigners' who drop in from the university, and are not seen as being remote from practice by agency staff.

The role also includes some lecturing and tutoring. This varies as a component of the total role, but its inclusion is of much importance. Were formal teaching sessions restricted to full-time lecturers only, clinical teaching could be interpreted as being of less importance. To registered nurses who have spent much of their nursing life educating patients on a one-to-one basis or in a group situation, however, facing a group of up to one hundred and fifty nursing students for the first time in the lecture setting can be an unnerving experience. Although staff receive some in-service training in classroom skills, teaching and learning theories are only superficially covered. The preparation alone seems to take up so much time initially. In addition, there is that inbuilt fear that the lecturer is responsible for ensuring that the students receive everything they need to know, so the preparation must be exhaustive, as the following excerpt shows.

I remember the work that was involved in giving my first lectures. It took days and days of searching through the library, reading and writing and rewriting notes for the first lecture. Overheads had to be produced expertly and I had no idea how to make them look professional, not to overcrowd the page and to only contain the relevant points. The content of the lecture had to be specific and I had to know precisely when to use the overhead and to remember to switch it off at the right time, and more importantly how to time the delivery so that I used all the allotted time, no less and no more.

I was terrified when the day came. I arrived early and ran into an experienced lecturer whom I had known for many years. We chatted casually and I mentioned that I was giving my first lecture today. He wished me good luck which was much appreciated and then I was on my own with 150 student nurses. I didn't seem to be able to move like experienced lecturers move, I just stood there and give them the 'goodies'.

After it was over I felt so relieved, somewhat satisfied, a little more confident but aware that I had such a lot to learn about teaching. (Hanna, 1988)

It is only through time and experience that confidence grows in facing a large group of students in a huge lecture theatre. Being exposed to different teaching styles as a tertiary student is helpful in developing a style which is most suitable for the individual. Receiving feedback, either from an experienced lecturer or through student evaluation, helps future teaching sessions. Despite that, there is always the fear that because you are not 'qualified' as an educator you may be doing a disservice to the students.

There are various schools of thought on this issue. One school believes that obtaining formal education in teaching is essential in order to teach effectively, whereas another school maintains that formal teacher training is not necessary, that knowledge embedded in expertise can be transmitted despite the lack of educational theory (Benner, 1984). It seems such a responsibility knowing that your part must be good, as the students only have a limited time in each subject area.

Tutorials seem far less threatening. For one thing, the size of the group is more manageable and one is more than likely to get to know the students more personally. There is a sense that students feel more comfortable with a regular, familiar face who can share with them the day-to-day goings on of the real world of nursing. It follows that the practitioner is dealing with current clinical issues on a daily basis and has a 'feel' for what nursing life is all about. In addition, the subject matter is usually not new to students, and open discussion is encouraged. To the student, the clinician/

lecturer is seen as credible, having come from recent clinical practice and therefore they are more likely to accept some things that are said to them. Despite that, considerable preparation time is needed and this is often only achieved by working in your own time.

The role with health agencies

Negotiating clinical placements for students with health agencies, whether they be hospital or community agencies, can be a particularly frustrating aspect of the job. It is the responsibility of the team organizing each nursing subject to find sufficient, appropriate placements for the students. Clinician/lecturers, being the link between clinical practice and the university, are often delegated this unenviable task. However, their special understanding of health agencies and knowledge of the quality of nursing care practised there makes them the most suitable people to undertake such a role.

With such large groups of students, it is a phenomenal task to find sufficient placements, let alone meaningful experiences for the students. In addition, there are unspoken geographical boundaries and fierce competition for student places, and we never dare 'poach' placements from outside our region. Initially, clinician/lecturers explore the region to find all the suitable agencies. Contact is then made personally with an agency staff member to discuss the school philosophy, the curriculum and more specifically the requirements for that particular subject. In many cases, approval cannot be given until Board of Management discussions take place. Once approval is granted, finer details have to be worked out regarding mode of dress, hours, matters concerning insurance and liability and any other specific requirements. The university then draws up legal contracts with agencies. The entire process sometimes takes months to finalise. As placement and agency agreements become established, arrangements can be repeated and a maintenance role develops rather than that of complex negotiation. Thus the pressure experienced in the initial stages of setting up courses lessens considerably over time.

Some units within the curriculum are more easily managed than others, in that only one or two hospitals are needed to accommodate the students. Other units are less fortunate, sometimes having to deal with anything up to seventy agencies. As can be imagined, explaining the university requirements over and over again becomes a less attractive part of the role, even though clinician/lecturers share this task. Not only is it incredibly time consuming running all around the region, but often the tertiary system has to be defended against well-intentioned nurses who believe that the students are not mature enough, or suitably experienced to deal with the day-to-day occurrences in any one agency.

Despite the teething problems, the integration of university students became less of a problem as time passed and staff began to accept the changing image of nursing. Having been practitioners for many years and well indoctrinated into the cultural norms of hospital practice, it is refreshing to have daily ward routines questioned and criticized by these young people, unexposed to the biases that the experienced practitioner develops over the years. The following journal excerpt indicates this well:

> Having left students on a ward one day to participate in shift handover, I returned later to find them confused and angry as to the way this routine ward procedure had been handled. Subjective, derogatory descriptions of clients had included such words as 'complainer', 'difficult', 'needs to try harder', and were interspersed by personal details of clients which were irrelevant and unrelated to their care. The students were puzzled as to why nurses as professionals had spoken of people under their care in such a fashion. It certainly did not fit with the image they had of nurses as carers. I did not have the answers. In fact I had heard so many handovers given this way over the years that I had stopped hearing this happen. The issues were discussed with the students, including reasons why staff may have lost sight of their objectivity. I also spoke to ward staff about it who were initially quite defensive. However, there has been a change in handover when students are participating. Although there is guardedness only when students are around to listen, perhaps in the future eventually all handovers will be handled with more sensitivity and objectivity. (Peart, 1990)

Such an example serves to suggest that for the clinician/lecturer not only is there a great deal to show and teach pre-registration students but there is always something refreshingly obvious to learn from them as well. The simple questions that students often ask, serve to make clinician/lecturers question many practices that had formerly been taken for granted. The students' receptivity to new ideas, their constructive comments and criticisms, highlight the circular benefits of promoting cooperation between clinician/ lecturers and students. In community agencies practitioners had differing and varied expectations to which students should be exposed as the following excerpt indicates;

> I felt very disappointed when a senior community nurse refused to take students on home visits, suggesting that they were too inexperienced and would have difficulty coping with some of the situations. She felt the students were too young and had little life experiences.
>
> In another situation, one young male student spent a day with a community health nurse in a rural area after which he delightfully related his experiences to the group during a formal de-briefing session. As the philosophy of the school is based on reflection in and on practice, these sessions formed a valuable part of their day to day experiences and were able to be put in context by the experienced practitioner. The young student was amazed to find such old, filthy houses, without the expected modern facilities, to find 'black things in the bath', which his fellow students hilariously said were leeches, to be given instructions by the nurse not to accept a drink in a specific house because of the level of hygiene. He also described the rural 'grapevine', which heralded their pending arrival from one house to the next, and the wonderful community spirit where people helped each other. (Hanna, 1990)

It is those experiences that stand out in a student's mind which provide rich learning opportunities and material for discussion, irrespective of what they are up to in their education.

An interesting problem arose in the area of community health. Health agencies wanted to know exactly what we required the students to do, and in some situations wanted learning objectives. The faculty prefers a process curriculum whereby students are required to negotiate what they want to learn, which presented a problem for agencies. Where the agency employed nurses on the staff, it was made easier, but the students needed broader experiences and therefore health agencies were used which did not employ nurses. We wanted the students to experience such areas as social services, dental health, meals on wheels, home help, health education and community education amongst others. We found it difficult to specify tasks for the students to do, recognizing that each agency offered unique experiences. Agencies felt that because they were not providing nursing care, they had nothing to offer the student. It took considerable discussion to convince them that nurses did more than tasks. The students also needed reminding of this, many of them feeling disappointed in the lack of 'real' nursing in their first year.

A further practical problem was encountered in negotiating suitable days. Students were restricted to specific days owing to the nature of the course. Some agencies were only available on specific days, whereas others were only available once a fortnight or once a month. It became a nightmare to juggle names, agencies and days while taking into consideration student requests, lack of private transport and their geographical location. It was a wonderful feeling when all the discussions were over and placements were allocated.

Throughout clinical placements, clinician/lecturers are responsible for students. In hospitals, clinician/lecturers work alongside students, while in the community they visit the students in various settings. Ongoing contact with agency staff is essential throughout the duration of, and following the placement. This way, difficulties can be ironed out and we are more likely to be successful in achieving ongoing high quality experiences for the following year. Good communication skills are a prerequisite and discussions with staff in the agencies is an ongoing process, since there are always staff changes, policies changes, management changes and philosophy changes.

Advantages and challenges

One of the major challenges experienced by clinician/lecturers is the merging of roles. Multiple roles of nurse, teacher and student within the space of one day can be both physically and emotionally draining. A sense of identity becomes rather confusing as the various roles demand different behaviours and approaches from the nursing perspective. In many instances the dual role of clinician/lecturer can leave the nurse feeling like the 'meat between the sandwich' when it comes to satisfying both the faculty's educational and practical requirements for its pre-registration students while at the same time ensuring the hospital's or health agencies' protocols and routines are adhered to. The need to be totally committed to all these areas can leave one with a sense of inadequate preparation or a feeling of having completed no one task satisfactorily owing to the heavy workload involved;

> Yet there is a positive side to the role of clinician/lecturer or why would I still be doing it. It has led to personal growth within my own practice as a nurse, professional growth in my quest to pursue further study, and an overall feeling of being part of something worthwhile. The multiple roles, while exhausting, have broadened my understanding of practice and certainly returning to student status myself has given me a better understanding of stressors young pre-registration students must try and deal with. (Peart, 1990)

For some people, multiple roles can be very time consuming. The pressures of personal and family life may become enormous, and family life may become slotted in around the diverse challenges of the role. This is not always evident to anyone outside the family as each component of the clinician/lecturer role can be perceived as part-time to an outsider. These part-time roles inevitably add up to a considerable number of hours, often making more than a normal full-time job. Yet as a part-time worker in more than one role, there may be a feeling that one does not quite belong anywhere.

Working within two very different systems does not necessarily mean that hours worked in agencies are evenly spaced which can lead to extra demands.

> I am always tired. I work ten hours in delivery suit on Friday, Saturday and Sunday and catch a few hours sleep before coming back at 1 pm on Mondays only to be back again by 7 am Tuesday. In the meantime there are journals to be read for the students and tutorial preparation to be done before Friday. Somewhere in between I have to study my own course. There are precious few hours for family life. It is no wonder my husband gets cross. He hasn't seen me for a week. (Peart, 1990)

For would-be clinician lecturers it is important to be able to integrate all roles into a lifestyle without too much disruption to personal or family life.

Challenges in the clinical setting include coping with the 'horizontal violence' of workmates who will never accept that there could be different or better ways of educating student nurses. Negative stereotyping of other nurses, particularly student nurses, is a widespread and commonly practised behaviour, which, it has been argued, is inherent behaviour amongst oppressed groups (Roberts, 1983). Roberts argues that nurses as members of such a group manifest similar traits found in other oppressed groups. Nurses view themselves negatively and develop a fatalism which rejects evidence to the contrary in order to maintain and perpetuate the accepted myths (Street, 1990). Although this makes the clinician's job as an intermediary more difficult, it is so refreshing to work with young people who remain unaffected by such stereotypes.

Working with students is a positive learning experience in that it makes the clinician think seriously about many things taken for granted in practice. Their simple, sometimes obvious, questions may reflect the way many clients can see a nurse in action, and leave no doubt that sometimes there is room for improvement. Not all their comments are critical. Student nurses are quick to recognize the intuitive skills of the experience practical nurse who seems to be in control of all situations no matter how distressing. Unanimously they seem amazed at the nurse's ability to organize a myriad of duties and details within a short space of time. Not only do students see flaws with the systems, they also marvel at skills and expertise which they feel sure they will never master.

Frustration in the academic setting stems from the clinician's own perceived inexperience in teaching. Dealing with difficult, disruptive, sometimes unmotivated students requires somehow acquiring teaching strategies to keep them interested. A further difficulty arises between agencies and academic staff because of the limited time spent at university by the clinician. As a result, problems arise in organizing sufficient and appropriate placement for students with agencies so that students somehow get some sort of meaningful experience.

Despite the difficulties there is an opportunity for the clinician to participate in changing what nurses read, think, talk about, write about, and do about nursing. That is exciting and challenging. That is what represents the very positive role of being a clinician/lecturer – being a change agent.

The opportunity to interact with visiting nursing scholars who represent the thoughts of many international colleagues, and to exchange ideas and ways of improving what nurses have to offer society is of great advantage to the practice-orientated clinician. National and international gurus become available for university staff to exchange thoughts and ideas. The humanness of this exchange and the desire of these people to make nursing something better leaves those new to academia feeling overwhelmed but encouraged for the future of nursing.

Reflection on the role

Being clinician/lecturers has had a marked effect on us as nurses. There is no doubt that further study has caused us to think differently, but sometimes it is hard to know whether these benefits have come from our personal study or whether they have been derived from our role as clinician/lecturers.

We have become so defensive about the programme. Nurses who went through the hospital training system and who have made no attempt to update their nursing knowledge are continually attacking the tertiary system. They cannot understand why nurses need a theory-laden course compared with their apprentice style programme. Comments are continually made regarding the students' immaturity, lack of motivation, lack of knowledge, lack of practical skills and so forth. Being at the interface between university and agency allows many of these questions to be answered and acted upon before problems arise. Having clinician/lecturers in many agencies throughout the nursing community ensures that both agency and student needs are taken into consideration.

Nursing academics often have a very positive outlook on nursing. Questioning why we do what we do is encouraged and change is actively pursued. Being part of a team that want only for nurses to reach their fullest potential and is keen for the profession of nursing to improve its knowledge base can only enhance a clinician's expertise.

We have also had to defend our positions on many occasions.

'Why put yourself through such an ordeal?' we are asked. What do you hope to gain? Where do you expect it to lead? Why do further study when you already have a good job? Do you want to become a full-time academic as a result? It is hard to explain that what we are doing is right for us. We have gained so much ourselves and this is reflected in the number of enquiries or consultations we have had with experienced nurses regarding a variety of nursing issues, who acknowledge our changed role.

Being clinician/lecturers has led us into continuing education and caused us to become academically curious. It has enhanced our own personal growth and professional development and raised many questions in our minds. For one of us, some of these questions have culminated in a funded research project, an area that would have been otherwise unexplored. This was made possible by being a staff member which brings with it perks such as using the expertise of experienced researchers, and having access to university research funds which would not normally have been available.

We do not profess to be experts, but to our fellow workers, we are familiar and approachable people who may be able to answer their questions or suggest where answers may be obtained. Throughout the experience, we have managed to influence other nurses in their practice, by raising issues they may be unable to see. In addition, some nurses have been encouraged to explore the area of further study themselves, and this is a rewarding outcome.

We are unaware whether we meet the ideals set by the faculty. The demands are great. The ability to give total commitment to every facet of our varied roles is questionable. We seem to work very hard yet often feel frustrated with not being able to give more, but there are only so many hours in the day.

The benefit of hindsight

What would make nurses more prepared for a multifaceted role such as that of a clinician/lecturer? Perhaps a thorough orientation and exploration of the purpose of the university programme would be helpful. Sound leadership from experienced university lecturers is essential and even some hints on teaching strategies to lessen the newcomer's inexperience with students. Adequate time for planning of lectures and a workload congruent with the amount of time spent on campus would be helpful as ultimately the heavy workload will result in some degree of frustration and the need to prioritize.

Despite the challenges, the multiple roles of teacher, nurse and student have affected our practice of nursing and our own personal philosophies and beliefs in a very special way. Changes no longer seem so impossible. We no longer accept the argument that 'it has always been done this way so it must be right'. We find ourselves advocating patients' rights and not allowing ourselves to be intimidated by other staff members as the following excerpt shows:

> I had never challenged a doctor like that before but I knew he was not giving the complete story. I felt I had to say something – not to let him get away with this. So I challenged him, fairly nervously but confident in the accuracy of my information . . . I was thrilled, feeling as though I had achieved so much and it is only through incidents like this that we [nurses] will get anywhere with protecting the rights of individuals. (Hanna, 1988)

If the way we care for people is better, then all the challenges have been worthwhile. We have enjoyed the challenges and the obvious changes that have occured within ourselves and the way we practice as nurses. We will continue to explore further nursing issues through nursing students, our own research, study and practice. Learning never ceases, and we feel richer for the experience.

References

Benner, P. (1984) *From Novice to Expert: Excellence and Power in Clinical Nursing Practice.* Addison-Wesley, California

Deakin University (1988) *Diploma of Nursing Curriculum Document.* Deakin University, Geelong

Hanna, B. (1988–1991) Personal professional journal

Peart, K. (1990–1991) Personal professional journal

Roberts, S. (1983) Oppressed group behaviour: implications for nursing. *Advances in Nursing Science,* **5** (4), 21–30

Street, A. (1990) *Nursing Practice: High Hard Ground, Messy Swamps and the Pathway in Between.* Deakin University Press, Geelong

9

The joint appointment

Helen Cox, Barbara Hanna and Kerry Peart

Introduction

The people who occupied the joint appointee posts at the time this work was commissioned (Pauline and Shirley) have both moved on to new posts. Hence this chapter has been written by colleagues who worked with them at the time and is based on both formal interviews and informal discussions about their experiences in the role. Nevertheless it offers a vivid description of both the joys and the difficulties of working in this way.

The joint appointment model is not a new concept, having been tried both in the United Kingdom and in the United States of America with varying degrees of success. The literature indicates that establishing such roles has not been an easy task. This particular model involves two registered nurses who, between them, make up one full-time charge nurse and one full-time lecturer. The charge nurse position is located in a Professorial Nursing Research Unit which has, as its focus, extended care and rehabilitation. The unit is part of a large regional centre that cares for more than six hundred elderly residents with varying levels of dependence and independence. The lecturer position is with the Faculty of Nursing in the university, and involves chairing two units of study (subjects) within the pre-registration Bachelor of Nursing Course, one unit in each of the two semesters (terms). Unit Chairpersons are responsible for the planning, implementation and evaluation of the units of study as they contribute to the overall programme and progression of students through the course.

A major aim in establishing joint appointments between clinical agencies and educational institutions is to address the so-called 'gap' between theory and practice; between education and service. Wright (1988) reminds us of how easy it is to locate evidence of situations where the practical experience of student nurses fails to match the ideals with which they are imbued in the classroom. This has the dual effect of disillusionment for students and reduction in the quality of care that patients receive. How often do we as clinicians say, or as teachers hear 'that is how they tell you to do it "over there", but let me show you how it is really done here!'. A registered nurse with feet solidly planted in the realities of both worlds sounds like an ideal solution to a timeless dilemma.

An assumption implicit in the joint appointment concept is that the registered nurse who is also a teacher will bring to the clinical setting rich and exciting innovations and up-to-date ideas derived from research. Another assumption is that the practitioner who is also a teacher will bring to the educational setting a grasp of the real world of nursing, with its 'grass roots' practical issues, thus preventing the decline into 'ivory tower academia' that nurses seem to perceive and fear occurring.

Can it work?

Serious cautionary notes have been raised about the viability of joint appointee roles. One aim of this section is to provide an honest appraisal of the situation as it exists, and to explore what has supported, and what has constrained the incumbents in their struggles to create a role which 'works'.

Kuhn (1982) makes a point which coincides with our own experience and is one factor which has driven our entire staffing profile; students know when they are being taught by people without credibility. This includes being taught about decision making in nursing by people who do not make nursing decisions; being taught about nursing procedures by people who never perform them; and observing teaching staff relating to nursing staff on wards as though they were visitors rather than team members.

The role: expectations and realities

A view held by staff in this faculty, and many others, refutes the idea that theory is somehow better and more worthy than practice, and that practitioners do not theorize. What is being achieved by the role of the joint appointment is the 'forging of a new road' (Wright, 1988) which rejects the assumptions of superiority of theory over practice and replaces it with the recognition of the 'interpenetration of the two' (Smyth, 1987).

Joint appointees have the potential to challenge the way things are and to effect changes in their practice setting, changes in their educational setting and indeed changes in themselves and those around them. As Wright suggests, it is clearly a business of 'role creation'.

The faculty considered that the role of joint appointment was potentially the most difficult of the three models being used. In recognition of this it was thought that having two people sharing both roles would provide an inbuilt support mechanism. The arrangement was that the two people would make up one charge nurse position in the one ward, rather than splitting them across different wards. Both people would also make up the one lecturer position, in the one unit of study. Thus one person would work two and a half days in the ward and the remainder of the week in the university and the other would do the opposite. The university calendar was able to provide a degree of flexibility that was not possible for a ward to provide, so a half day from the university portion was able to be spent occasionally on the unit allowing both incumbents to spend time planning and working together. Later a model of working a 'semester about' was tried where one joint appointee would spend the teaching weeks of the semester at the university, returning to the ward on Thursdays for faculty practice, but in the capacity of charge nurse. This one day each week ensured the maintenance of relationships with the residents and staff, and an ongoing contribution to planning within the unit. The other joint appointee would spend the teaching weeks on the ward, coming to the university on Thursdays to plan for the oncoming semesters teaching. This model had no overlap in the teaching weeks, but the university once again was able to provide some flexibility outside this time (there are twenty-two non-teaching weeks each year) so that the main planning could be done. Time will tell which model proves to be most effective.

The joint appointees were able to decide personally whether contracts would be between themselves and the hospital, with charge nurse entitlements, or the university with lecturer entitlements. These incumbents both chose the latter, so the hospital component was based on a secondment for 50% of the time for which the hospital reimbursed the university financially. This approach solved the dilemma of having two masters. It also changed the relationship that the joint appointees had with the hospital authorities who were technically not their employers. It seemed to promote a collegial framework where matters can be dealt with by discussion between equals, rather than other approaches which are sometimes seen in relationships between charge nurses and administrators.

At the time that these incumbents took up appointment they were both looking for change and for new challenges. They had both gained expertise as clinicians with strong backgrounds in elderly care and extensive experience in leadership positions. Attending a conference on the subject of 'Bridging the Gap' had led to a curiosity and interest as speakers explained their roles and experiences as joint appointees. Thus when the position of joint appointment with the faculty was advertised both felt that it would be an excellent way of testing out some ideas that the conference had evoked. One (Pauline) had known about the role previously, and felt quite comfortable about her ability within the agency, but she was less confident about the university aspect. Her fear was not related to her ability, but to a suspicion that perhaps starting in two new roles would be too great a workload. People had told them both not to take the positions, saying 'it is a dreadful job'. However, they knew each other; had worked together previously and were confident that they could work together as a team. They managed to keep each other enthusiastic about the role in the hope that they would be appointed together and this hope was realized.

Initially Pauline and Shirley spent as much time together as possible, talking, planning and reinforcing each other's ideas. When asked what their fears were at that time, they could confidently say:

None, as far as the type of nursing is concerned. We knew that we were very experienced, suitably qualified and were confident about our abilities to work creatively as charge nurses in the Professorial Nursing Unit. However there was some concern that the workload would be too much and that we would not live up to the expectations of both parties. Maybe we would have wonderful ideas and not be able to carry them out.

Despite their concern, they both considered the extra dimension of the university with its student contact to be a welcome challenge. Wright (1988) mentions the need for the joint appointees to be highly skilled people in both clinical nursing and in teaching, with conflict management as a particular area of expertise. He suspects that of all the roles that we may explore in nursing, the joint appointment is potentially the most conflict laden one. That was certainly the warning issued to these two as they stepped out on the path of exploring the ramifications of the appointment.

Conflict in Wright's eyes stems from three main sources:

- Between roles, e.g. the nurse who is also a wife and a mother.
- Within the role, e.g. the nurse who is both a clinician and a teacher in the formal sense.
- In the role set, e.g. the perceptions people have about the role and what it entails.

Pauline and Shirley have experienced all three sources of conflict, but the area of emphasis for them was the third, particularly in terms of the expectations that they would create change.

A vision of change

The notion of the joint appointee as a change agent was, in reality, a difficult aspect. They found themselves very busy as they moved into two independently demanding roles. They knew that the future would be challenging as they would be expected to create change. This was what they wanted and intended to do . . . but in the meantime they had to keep a twenty-five bed unit functioning smoothly.

Both Pauline and Shirley recognized and understood the implications of change and were particularly keen not to move too quickly. They were aware that change can be threatening, often causing staff members to wonder about what they had been doing wrong. Indeed, the aim of the joint appointee was to recognize and value the experience and expertise of the clinicians with whom they had been working.

Change needed to be introduced slowly and it was essential that everyone was clear about how that could be done. Many hours were spent deliberating about the best ways to work with people who were threatened, and who possibly did not understand the nature of a Professorial Nursing Unit. The task required a great deal of tact and diplomacy.

The perceptions of the residents were just as important. In fact they appeared to be very comfortable and it would have been quite wrong to start by saying that their world was going to be turned upside down. It was acknowledged that there was a need to work with the staff to develop a shared perception of what the possibilities could be. Careful explanations of the purpose of the new roles in the Professorial Nursing Unit were given, stressing that they were to explore and generate creativity and innovation in practice – not to identify what was bad, but constantly to search for ways in which it could be bettered.

In the end it was decided that nothing would be done, quite deliberately, for the first three months, but to watch, listen, think and talk about possibilities. Staff and residents knew that this was the plan, having been included in all tentative discussions.

Talks also took place about the need to consider the effects of the changes which would be introduced in terms of industrial conditions. Changes usually influence people's working lives and conditions in some way. It was considered important to conduct discussions with staff other than the nurses themselves, as the changes to routines would impact on people such as kitchen staff, cleaning staff, and others. There was also a need to discuss proposals with union representatives.

One particular example of negotiating change with ancillary staff occurred over the matter of residents having the right to have breakfast in bed if they wished. This had clear implications for the kitchen staff, but when consulted in a general discussion, their attitude was 'why not, it's what I like when I feel tired or a bit unwell'. Including the ancillary staff in all discussions created a new sense of involvement, and it changed their relationships with the residents. They were not distanced, but felt intrinsic to the running of this unit. Morale and a sense of involvement amongst staff seemed almost like a substitute for a family. This was exactly the environment which it had been hoped could exist in what was really these people's home.

Staff work on the unit on the basis of having applied and been selected. They are there because they want to be, and their level of commitment to the goals of the unit are high. There is a strong sense of wanting to be part of changes in nursing practice that serve the best interests of the residents. Everyone shared a desire to explore the possibilities and dimensions of the joint appointee role which could bring about such things.

Creating change often takes some courage. One story about a doctor doing a round with medical students serves to demonstrate this point. This particular doctor went to a patient who was sitting in the day room and proceeded to lift her dress and explain about her knee condition to his students. This was such an unusual occurrence in the unit that the nurses went quickly to seek out one of the joint appointees. The unit has a policy that if a resident requires a doctor, a request is made in the same manner as someone asking for a home visit. In this instance it was Pauline who went quickly and quietly to ask the resident if the doctor had asked her permission to examine her knee; not only did she say 'no', but she was red faced and indignant, saying 'what a cheek!'. The doctor was then reminded gently that this was not the type of ward that he was used to but was more like a home for the residents. He was asked if he would remember to consult with the nurse should he visit the ward again. The message in this experience was not the apparent lack of concern for the resident's feelings, but the assumptions that were made about the relationship between doctors and residents in health agencies. There was no malicious intent, simply a way of being and doing that had developed, without examination, over time. To his credit, next time this doctor wanted to bring students to hear 'an interesting chest I believe you have down there' he rang and asked permission. The staff were able to say 'just a moment and I will ask Mrs X if she would like you to examine her'. On checking with Mrs X she said that she did not want to see them. That was that! This type of assertiveness from staff takes experience and maturity, but it also takes courage.

There have been other instances where doctors have had to make adjustments in the way they work with, and perceive, both the nurses and the residents. At one time there was a doctor who was holding tightly to being the power broker in the unit, intervening in what were clearly nursing matters. Pauline and Shirley were able to gently challenge this and were successful to the point that the doctor eventually asked how she could help in the management of residents in the unit . . . what did the nurses wish her role to be? After that she came when requested, discussed problems in a collegial manner, including the resident as well as listening to the advice of those who were familiar with the resident's problems and wishes. The entire manner of interaction was changed to a more professional level.

Through many years of professional experience in senior positions, both the joint appointees have developed the ability to challenge inappropriate behaviour in what they hope are helpful ways. One example involved the nursing handover, where some quite subjective and often inappropriate things were being said. This is a theme that was encountered earlier in this chapter but in this case the joint appointees were in a position to challenge the behaviour 'from the inside'. One of them (whoever was around at the time) would stop the handover and ask what had prompted the remark, not so much as to berate the speaker, but to examine the underlying irritation or belief that gave rise to the comment. The staff moved from defensiveness, to justification, to self critique and finally to a new richness in how they perceived the situation. Through acting as role models themselves the joint appointees started to empower other staff and through them the residents.

Supports and constraints to the change agency role of the joint appointment

Having two registered nurses who share two roles is perhaps more likely to succeed than where individuals have two halves to their role without sharing the same roles. The mutuality in the concept is supportive and sustaining. The single most important feature in making the role a success is the compatibility between the two incumbents. It seems to require a level of maturity that has moved beyond competing. From the experience of these two joint appointees it can be suggested that the critical factor is selecting the right people to work so closely together.

It is recognized that many other factors impact on the success or otherwise of the role, not least of which is the committed team of registered and enrolled nurses on the unit, all of whom offered support in different ways. There is no doubt that their personalities are also a key feature in the success or otherwise of what the joint appointees strive to achieve.

Another finding was that the environment which was fostered promotes retention of staff who find it meets their need to give a high quality of care. There is a clear feeling of pride which is reflected by a sentiment which is common in the team:

> If it was my own mum, and she was elderly and in need of care, I would feel quite happy that she was in this unit.

Flexibility was another feature that was found to be both supportive and constraining. As was said earlier, it is not always possible to have flexibility in the unit, because the residents are always there and in need of care. But from the university side, the students are not always there, and there are times when the course planning is up to date, the clinical placements are set up and it is possible to spend more time together planning for things on the unit. Sometimes in intersemester (term) breaks, each of the incumbents work half a week each and overlap a bit, which also gives them more time in each area.

Time is an enemy, as it has been with each model described in this chapter. One of the joint appointees (Shirley) had been a clinician/lecturer previously and found that hard enough. It is a lot harder to be a joint appointee. As her journal reflects:

> It is terribly difficult, you feel that you have got to be giving both halves of the job sufficient time and yet you end up giving both halves more time than one full job. It is very hard work. Whether with practice it becomes better . . .?

In the early days a whole semester would go by when no study leave could be taken, despite efforts being made to find the time. Both Pauline and Shirley were also studying and striving for the success they felt was needed in their roles. Lack of time was indeed a hardship, however the common feeling was that they could not do things by halves. Maybe this says something about the degree of commitment they both felt for their work which may be a prerequisite for roles such as theirs. It is clear that these models are problematic if one wishes to maintain a thirty-eight or forty hour week but some incumbents have seen this same time management issue as a challenge to be overcome.

Further to this notion of two halves of the job is another insidious problem; the fact that no one sees you in any full-time capacity. An assumption can be made that you are only working part time, and hence are not as busy . . . having the easy life!

At the time these were the only joint appointees in Victoria. They had no colleagues in similar roles with whom to relate and share troubles and triumphs. This makes the joint appointment a potentially lonely role. It underscores the intense need for two people in the role and for strong support from staff in both institutions.

Sometimes they got the feeling that others did not appreciate the complexity of the work:

A feeling in this agency that anyone can do this if they have the kind of residents that they perceived that we had. They didn't really need any nursing care and that sort of thing. I felt compelled to look after people who needed a higher level of care just so that we could say 'we can still run this unit as we want to and we have the same sort of people as you'. I remember someone saying to me 'you don't have to prove anything to them, but I still had this feeling that we did'. Some RNs were threatened and resentful, they would nitpick and write sarcastic comments in the communication book. (Shirley)

Reflecting on this anecdote, we have pondered whether it points out a fundamental problem in the use of communication books – that they may promote distance and more oblique communication rather than face-to-face resolution of issues.

However, Pauline and Shirley found ways of coping with such things. When they found themselves getting really upset, they sat down and talked to the staff member concerned about it, suggesting that the comments were inappropriate. They found that this was often effective and gave others a chance to gain some insight into their roles.

Extended time away from the ward can also bring both joys and worries. One incident which was recalled was concerned with a time when Shirley had been absent for a while and on visiting the unit one day found new furniture installed. Staff had been out to select lounge suites which were placed around the day room. While this added to the appearance of comfort and homeliness on the unit, it brought with it a pang. As Shirley said:

> all these things are happening and it has got nothing to do with me . . . it is not that I feel that I have lost control, but it has been a long time since I have had a significant input into the Unit.

This feeling arose because Shirley was the one spending four days each week at the university and only one on the unit. Even though she visited the unit at the end of the clinical days she spent with students, this did not seem enough. It was difficult to keep that feeling of belonging.

However there is also an 'up side' to this story. When work was started on the unit none of the staff would have felt the energy or drive to take such an initiative without asking permission. Indeed it is unlikely that they would have even thought of it. In a relatively short space of time there had been a significant change in attitude.

Although the clinical component of their role was satisfying and they were confident that they were achieving their goals, in the early days both Pauline and Shirley were unsure about their university role. Sharing the semester had its problems and each found certain new responsibilities more difficult than expected. The early model, where roles were swapped half way through the week, was confusing for the students. They were uncertain who would be present to run their tutorials or to supervise their clinical practice. Because the joint appointees had differing personalities, students did not know how to 'read' them in order to feel confident about responses they were preparing. In addition, occasionally the person who discussed assessments would not be the person who conducted them. Students felt that they were not well served by the arrangement. This was, in part, the stimulus for the move to swap roles each semester rather than at the mid-week point.

Working with students at their own agency, even though it was not always in their own ward, was excellent. As far as the staff's perception of them as charge nurse and as a facilitator of students was concerned there were barriers at first. But over time a lot of these barriers were broken down and they felt that the students were accepted more readily; that the RNs realized that they were not just people with 'airy fairy' ideas; that they were able to do basic practical common sense nursing; and that students were learning that too.

Reflections

Both Pauline and Shirley have tried to reflect on whether they have lived up to everyone's expectations, let alone their own. To a certain extent the answer is 'yes'. Not long ago they had that feeling that they really had not been able to do very much which led them to sit down together to work out just what had been achieved. It was not until a report was written for the Professor and the agency that they came to realize how much they had actually accomplished.

There had been changes to routines, staffing, structures and processes, and to relationships. That does not mean that there are no routines now, but they are the routines which residents like to have observed. Similarly some tasks are important and there are always activities which simply have to be done each day. The difference is a change of emphasis from rituals and routine for their own sake.

The joint appointees have also wondered how much influence they have had on nurses and nursing within the agency. Although there was some initial wariness, this has receded with time. Colleagues seem more relaxed and comfortable about referring people. Comments such as

> what do you think about Mrs so and so, she is rehabilitating really slowly, but we would like to think that she could continue with her rehabilitation, what do you think about taking her on to the Unit?

are becoming common practice.

Another positive outcome of the arrangement between the university and the agency is an increased interest in nursing education. It is hard to see just who and what influenced such change but it is happening in pockets everywhere. It appears that the joint appointees may well have contributed by acting as role models, and by doing some 'in service' lectures and group discussions. Some of the nurse scholars visiting the university have also given seminars and conferences for the staff. Similarly students are taken through the unit for in-service development and they share ideas and ideals. All of this is helpful and influential and may have played a part in promoting this positive view of nurse education.

One thing which both Pauline and Shirley think is important is that they can recognize the need to seek expert help from other nurses where relevant. An example of this appeared in another anecdote:

> There was a woman who was exhibiting periods of psychotic behaviour, we had some discussion about whether she ought to be transferred to the psychogeriatric unit. We didn't want to do that, we have the attitude that this was her home. We asked the nurses in the psychogeriatric ward to assess her, and then to help us with her management. With their help she settled down again and we were able to manage her quite successfully without moving her out. We had to do something, because the others were getting upset, and it is their home too.

Another important message in this example is that help was not sought from a psychiatrist, but from expert psychiatric nurse practitioners.

Pauline and Shirley know that they have both similarities and differences. They were similar in hopes, aspirations and philosophies as far as the residents and the unit were concerned but not similar in personality. One was more 'up front', saying what was in her mind, whereas the other one was quieter, deliberating before responding. It may be that the dissimilarity allowed them to relate together so well in a complimentary fashion.

They both enjoyed the role of joint appointee – it turned out better than they had anticipated. They both learnt so much more about themselves as nurses, and as people, though they had to 'fine tune' their negotiation and diplomacy skills. They say that they have re-energized their spirit of enquiry, and their interest levels are recharged through the double challenge.

Steve Wright ends his paper with an invitation to institutions considering joint appointments, 'proceed by all means – but with caution'. We would add to this our own note – 'be cautious by all means, but choose the joint appointees wisely and invest both your total support and your trust'.

Pauline Donnelly is now practising in New South Wales.
Shirley Maloney is now working as a nurse researcher at Deakin University.

References

Kuhn, J. (1982) An experience with a joint appointment. *American Journal of Nursing*, **82**(**10**), 1570–1571
Smyth, W. J. (1987) *A Rationale for Teachers' Critical Pedagogy: A Handbook*. Deakin University Press, Geelong
Wright, S. (1988) *What is a Joint Appointment*. Bridging the Gap Conference Proceedings, Deakin Institute of Nursing Research, Geelong

Part Four
Alternative approaches

Lecturer practitioners and the various forms of joint appointment as portrayed in the previous chapters offer particular approaches to unified roles, or the bringing together of the different functions such as education, practice and management. Further, the examples described so far show the centrality of practice in nursing. They demonstrate how clinical settings, by the efforts of innovative practitioners who are visionary and analytical, staff and students can be educated and developed *and* high quality care can be facilitated.

Such conditions feature in other situations also. For example, a variant of the joint appointment is that of job sharing, where two people set out to occupy one role, in this instance that of ward sister for a medical ward, and Nursing Development Units can be viewed as clinical environments where practice and practitioners alike are changing and being changed for the ultimate benefit of improved patient care.

Judith Lathlean, having undertaken an evaluation of an earlier job share arrangement (Lathlean, 1987), and recognizing the potential for bringing theory and practice together in this role, extensively interviewed one of the job occupants together with her new partner. Her interpretation of their job – checked out by the partners – is presented in Chapter 10. Job sharers promote the advantages of two people having joint authority and responsibilities that attach to one post, but with the opportunity to bring different expertise, skills and ideas to bear on the planning and implementation of the work, and the benefits of mutual support. However, job sharers are not without their problems and challenges, for example, the necessity for the individuals to be aiming for the same goals, the inevitability of compromise in some instances in the ways adopted to attain these goals, the importance of effective communication, and the need for support from the organization.

In the arrangement described here, the occupants decided that rather than both being equally involved in all aspects of the job of sister, they would trade on their special attributes and inclinations, and thus each had different priorities. Yet whilst they were able to reach an informal agreement to do this, and one that they felt seemed to work well, it was not always appreciated by the organization which had a particular view about the way things should be. This job share also had other ingredients that are relevant to the theme of this book; for example, it was evident that both partners believed in the notion of a unified role as the senior clinical role, and both consciously drew on their research interests and expertise in carrying out their clinical work, though one more overtly than the other.

Nursing Development Units (NDUs), whilst by no means new, are increasingly being used as the vehicle to focus emphasis on the development of advanced nursing practice, where experimentation in therapeutic nursing care is deliberately encouraged, facilitated and supported. Steve Wright in Chapter 11 describes them as places which attempt 'to bring people and ideas together, to provide a climate where learning and innovation flourish, and to provide settings where the goals of education can be coterminous with those of practice'. As such they make a 'potential contribution to narrowing the gap between the theory and practice of nursing'.

Finally, it is no coincidence that innovative practitioners in multifaceted roles, and developmental nursing environments are intertwined. For example, within the next two chapters alone, one of the job sharers came from an NDU, and her views were heavily influenced by it. Her partner, subsequent to the job share, has developed the medical ward into an NDU. Also, Steve Wright became the clinical nurse specialist for an NDU, having once been a joint appointee. In conclusion, these two contributions, in common with other chapters, must be seen as offering alternative but by no means mutually exclusive perspectives on the same theme – that of putting theory into practice and practice into theory.

Reference

Lathlean, J. (1987) *Job Sharing a Ward Sister's Post*. Ashdale Press, Peterborough

10

Job sharing

Judith Lathlean with Angela Heslop and Shelagh Sparrow

Introduction

Job sharing is still a relatively unusual phenomenon in a health care setting and especially with nursing posts. This chapter describes an arrangement whereby two nurses occupied one post – that of ward sister for a medical ward. In addition, both had other jobs within the hospital, one as a respiratory health worker (Angela Heslop) and the other as a nurse researcher (Shelagh Sparrow). In this way they jointly operated in clinical and research settings, and shared between them the responsibility for the management of one ward. Through this unique combination of managerial and clinical activities, and the opportunity for one to engage in research and the other to work in a complementary clinical role, they were able to bring research to bear on their practice, and develop their clinical area in partnership. As such this situation bears many similarities to the collegiate lecturer practitioner role described in Chapter 6.

The story related in this chapter has two aspects – that of the sharing of one job by two people and the notion of one person having a combined clinical, educative and research role, and the other a managerial, practice and educative function. In both respects, this has implications for theory and practice. But first, the arrangement is put in its context, the way in which it was planned to operate is described and then the implications, challenges, achievements and problems are outlined.

The background to the job share

Prior to the job share described here, Angela had a strong clinical, educational and managerial background, as well as previous research experience – evaluating the intervention of a nurse visiting patients with disabling chest disease in the community (Heslop and Bagnall, 1988) and, as part of a multidisciplinary team, investigating the psychotherapeutic management of patients with breathing problems (Rosser *et al.*, 1983). She had worked before with another sister in a similar job share within the same clinical area (Lempp and Heslop, 1987), and had valued the way in which, as she put it, they 'were able to bounce ideas off one another'. Indeed, in an evaluation of the previous job share (Lathlean, 1987), it was clearly identified as one of the benefits.

Having developed a respiratory nursing service, and wanting both to play a role in this and to continue with the ward sister job share, she specifically welcomed the opportunity to embark upon a new partnership, this time with a person who had particular clinical skills and expertise and a research orientation. She felt that this was likely to bring 'a further rich dimension to the clinical work'. Shelagh had worked as a clinical nurse specialist in research, but in this post missed being in clinical practice. She had a firm belief that 'as a researcher [she] needed to be clinically credible, since a lot of nursing research is not used because people think it is done in ivory towers, divorced from practice'. She had also practised as a primary nurse in a Nursing Development Unit where she had experienced the 'redundancy' of the traditional role of the ward sister, finding it to be more that of a coordinator of nursing staff, a resource and information provider and a support giver (Sparrow, 1986). She too welcomed the chance to have a full-time post which combined the elements of research nurse and work in a clinical environment where a forward looking ethos in relation to the management of patient care was already being promoted. For example, the previous job share arrangement had led to a reconceptualization of the ward sister role and a move towards a modified form of primary nursing for the ward.

The two people brought together vital skills and aspirations. As Angela indicated:

> Personally, I wanted to continue the job share because I thought we could develop primary nursing more with Shelagh's background.

It would use some of her theoretical understanding for nursing practice issues: by virtue of *who* she is, she brings a more scientific approach than I can. Because of her experience she has developed analytical skills – I am more managerial. But my management strengths, combined with her practice and research scrutiny, gave us authority.

The awareness of their mutual advantages and the ability to apply their joint knowledge and expertise were clearly important from the outset.

Developing the job

In terms of the job share, the expectation of the organization was that both partners would share the role of the ward sister for the medical ward and all its responsibilities. They agreed that the job had a number of components:

- A structural management role.
- The development of individual staff.
- Teaching and research.
- A clinical specialist function.

However, they challenged the notion that a traditional ward sister role was appropriate in a primary nurse setting, and the implications of this are explored later. Further, it very quickly became evident that Shelagh's expertise and inclination lay especially in clinical practice and the application of research to this, rather than in management as such. She described the feeling of being 'ground down' by certain management issues, and Angela confirmed how stressful this appeared to be for her colleague. Thus they made an informal agreement to change the job share, with Angela acting as the 'manager' for the ward, and Shelagh the 'researcher', but both being involved in the other aspects – teaching, staff development and clinical work.

It is interesting to see how their backgrounds influenced the way they went about their ward work. For example, Shelagh became 'a primary nurse *par excellence*', and in doing so 'attempted to avoid the conflict [for her] of engaging in management'. A large part of the job was looking at the nurses' planning of care, getting them to 'question their practice' and constantly asking the question 'why?'. In this she was consciously aware of trying to develop the nurses' practice and in turn the care of the patients, by being supportively analytical and at times drawing on her research knowledge and techniques. An example from Shelagh illustrates the interrelationship between practice and research, and also the effects it had on the different people involved:

> A lady was admitted with quite a severe pressure sore, and we decided to treat it with Granuflex. When the consultant saw it, it looked extremely yellow and pusey – as Granuflex does when it is removed. He immediately asked for a referral to a plastic surgeon, and ordered something that from my experience and the research evidence was unacceptable, and, in these circumstances, not beneficial to the patient. I was able to find the literature and point out the relevant parts to the medical staff, saying that these are the reasons why we don't feel this change is for the best, and that we *suggest* we might be on the right tack already. We were allowed to go ahead – and we recognised that this took courage on the part of the doctor.
>
> It did get better, and one of the means we used to show improvement was 'measurement'. Again, drawing on the relevant research, we selected the best tool and used it to measure the changes. This was 'proof' for the doctors, helpful for the patient (who, whilst unable to view the area herself, could see through the scores that her pressure sore was diminishing) and encouraging for the nurses. Now all wounds and pressure sores are measured.

In commenting upon these approaches, Angela summarized how Shelagh's presence 'helped to refine both the thinking about goals and about measurement'. She pointed out that the ward had always had this kind of orientation, but, as a professorial medical unit, the medical model of measurement had been dominant. Now it was proving possible to shift to a nursing focus for such activities.

Angela too had a specialist clinical practice role in that her expertise and work in the respiratory nursing service meant that she had considerable experience in, and an understanding generated through her research about the general needs of patients with chronic breathing problems. More precisely and equally important, she had specific knowledge of individual patients who moved between home and hospital.

Both were interested in promoting the better organization of nursing work. Shelagh was keen to 'encourage the ward to get away from routine and ritual', though in fact it was not as routinized as others in any case, and 'to develop patient-centred care as much as the organizational constraints allowed'. One outcome of this was a new system for the drugs trolley. After 'a great deal of effort' and 'some problems' they were finally able to move from having only one to two.

As Angela pointed out, changes such as these were not just about putting research into practice. They were also to do with 'making life easier for the individual nurses'. Organizational and developmental issues had always been her concern and interest. She explained what this meant for her, and the mutual roles of the partners in the process:

> We were not just interested in examining the practice, but also how nurses worked and what makes their working patterns better. The reward for the patient then in turn is that the nurse can do the job well. In the past, nurses were helpless – we, with our different contributions have been able to give them the power for such things, or the strength and capacity to change the way they work – or to argue and debate.

Both had a role in relation to student learning as well as in the development of the staff nurses. Though Shelagh did not specifically arrange to work with students – the primary and associate nurses were encouraged to do this since they were working on the ward on a daily basis – she did see it as important to consider the learning needs of the students and the part played by the ward in meeting these needs. In this respect one of the aspects that interested her particularly was that of the potential of the ward to inadvertently create dissonance for the students. She was aware that the students had enough conflict already as a result of 'the tourist notion of travelling around from ward to ward', without having their practice challenged as well – the approach she tended to adopt with the trained staff. Instead, she took a different tack, as demonstrated in the following example. This again shows the 'research thinking' that tended to permeate her practice:

> We were looking at the use of Mediswabs, and we had decided that there was no basis for using them when giving intra-muscular

injections. Again, this was not based on a hunch but on the evidence available. So what we then did was to explain the rationale behind it for the students, but we also said that they would probably be expected to use them on the next ward, and that they would have to make the decision for themselves. It's always difficult when policy and procedures say one thing, but the research is biased heavily in another direction. A lot of the policies we had were from the seventies, and they weren't based on research.

Another example of a difficulty she identified for the students was that of their knowledge of the newer ways of organizing nursing care. As she said:

The students' understanding of the nursing process and patient-centred practice was often not good when they came to us, so it meant continual teaching by everyone of what is meant, such as the importance of the written communication.

An aspect spanning organization and practice was that of ascertaining the dependency of patients and the implications that this had for nursing resources. Here Shelagh was able to use the work she was undertaking in her other role as nurse researcher for the hospital – the requirement to introduce dependency studies across the hospital. Because of her authority on this particular ward she was able to 'ensure that a system was looked at and put into place on the ward, with proper feedback'. In addition, she worked out 'a very crude grade mix analysis' which she hoped would help them to determine what mix of grades they needed, and also 'enable the staff nurses to have more clout when they knew dependency levels were high', another example of 'empowering' the nurses. Angela commented that these tools had proved to be very important since, and had been used and accepted as a justification for closing beds when resources dropped too far below dependency levels.

It was especially in respect of this and related areas of management work that the shared job was felt to be so vital. Both partners, because of their experience, very much felt that the usual role of ward sister was not right for this setting. As Angela explained:

In the past we have invested a lot on one person . . . usually the ward sister. We talk about the sister as the change agent, yet this is not always possible because that person will never have all the skills. Shelagh was able to do a lot of these things because of my management capacities. For example, she set up the skill mix and dependency work, and I made sure it was going to happen.

Nevertheless, both agreed that it was still important to have 'something in the shape of a ward sister' since registered nurses, especially when newly in post, cannot be expected to have *all* the skills and attributes – 'such as empathy, ethical awareness, the ability to describe and measure and to discuss and analyse' – that are necessary to manage even a small group of patients. With this belief, they set out 'to model the type of ward sister or senior nurse who should be managing a primary nursing group so that they are free to practice but are supported in this'.

Relationships between the job sharers

Much of the time of Angela and her partner in the previous job share was spent in working out the mutual roles and finding ways of truly sharing the job (Lathlean, 1987). Such activity was necessary in this job share too but seemed less dominant, possibly because the organization was now more used to such an arrangement, a great deal had been learnt from that experience, and the new partners were fairly clear about their contributions and interests.

As Shelagh pointed out, there needed to be realism in the partnership:

You can't actually be *one* person. Though we had very similar views on nursing, we had different backgrounds, skills and inclinations, so it was important to make the most of them.

Angela concurred with this, and added that their ways of going about the job were bound to differ, despite the interrelationships:

We had a similar professional commitment and goals, but we probably had different priorities. Mine were steeped in psychological, organisational issues and how learning might come through that, and Shelagh's were to do with analysis, research and learning. They clearly overlapped, and the different aspects should go hand-in-hand.

Importantly, they had constantly to plan and set targets together, and the atmosphere they were having to create and promote all the time was one of change. However, the benefits of having two people working on this appeared to have spin-offs for the staff. As Angela described:

> In our position, you have to have the vision to change and to push on with whatever the idea is, if you are to succeed. We found that by the duality the nurses learnt themselves. They see you always planning and targeting, and it is more obvious when two of you are doing it. Broadly speaking nurses tend not to do this normally, but it appeared that through observing us, they in turn were helped with their planning.

Interrelationships between the jobs

As mentioned before, both had other jobs apart from that of ward sister. Angela shared a post of respiratory health worker with another nurse, and together they represented the respiratory nursing service, which was funded by the community. She visited patients at home, and saw the same patients in hospital and the outpatient clinic, the rationale being that she could offer continuity of contact, and support their education in hospital, home and clinic. Because of the knowledge of patients in the various settings, she was able to give 'a very real picture of their needs and capabilities', and help to improve the quality of the goals of the patients. Thus, for example, because she was aware of the extent of Mr X's mobility in the hospital environment, and she knew the constraints of his home and surroundings, she could personally, or through others, work towards a realistic plan for his desired visit to the local library. And since she was knowledgeable about Mr Y's pride in growing his own yellow roses, she was able to suggest he had such roses when he died in hospital.

Indeed, in Angela's view it was this understanding of what it meant for a patient to be breathless, to go home, and to have to leave home and enter hospital that was both important to the quality of clinical care that she was able to provide, and her ability to pass the insight on to trained nurses and students. This was gained through her research and her work in the respiratory service. In turn this had benefits for her partner. As Shelagh said:

I had experience of organizing home visits but often through other people who were never available. It was so refreshing to have Angela who was able to bring the link back, and to explain to people that hospital was just one stage in people's lives. The social picture of patients was much easier to get.

Through this work, Angela was able to contribute 'formally and informally' to the learning of others about individual patients and about the care of patients with breathing problems. This was noted by Shelagh who said that it was very evident that students were able to relate the problems of breathlessness to all the activities of daily living (the basis of the model of nursing that was used on the ward). They did not just put in the notes 'has difficulty breathing' but would link it with a number of key aspects such as communication, the use of an oxygen mask, the effect on relationships and so on. Angela believed that with a combination of very formal teaching, and the powerful exemplars that she and the ward were able to provide, it enabled the students to learn, and hopefully to transfer this learning to 'seeing all patient care in a more person-centred way'.

She was also convinced that this had benefits for the trained staff and students alike in that they were 'no longer afraid of breathlessness', in part because it had been demonstrated fairly conclusively that 'you could do something about it, and that there were strategies to be employed which would make a difference'. This was also one of Angela's rationales for returning to the ward after having done the respiratory research. As she explained:

Armed with this knowledge, I wanted to see if I could make a difference to the nursing care of such patients. In this way both of my research projects have been fed back into the ward.

Shelagh's other role was that of research nurse for the hospital. One aspect of the work has already been mentioned, that of implementing dependency studies across the board, with the use of the ward to refine and implement it as well as possible. Another area of work was that of quality assurance, and it was hoped that 'innovative research' in this respect could be helpful within the hospital and especially in the ward. However, this proved to be a problem since the hospital was not particularly receptive to the ideas, maybe because research was not valued, and the fact that Shelagh had trained in the hospital and some found it difficult to accept her now well-developed research knowledge and expertise.

Indeed, the research role presented a number of difficulties. For example, though Shelagh's interest lay in being a research nurse, she was expected to set up a research unit with no obvious accommodation and with people who had little or no research experience, but in attempting to do so, this left little time for her to do research. Further, the two halves of her role were on different salary scales, and this caused some resentment amongst others. Added to which 'in [her] naivety', she had not negotiated a job description for the whole job, and thus there was lack of clarity and conflicts in expectations. This raised its own issues, and as Shelagh put it:

> The situation illustrated the dangers of not fitting into a hierarchy – people not knowing what to do with you, how to relate to you, and being resentful of your situation.

It appears that her research understanding and inclination were probably more influential in her work as a job-sharing ward sister than her hospital research nurse role, unlike Angela, where both her knowledge and the way her other role operated were helpful. In summarizing her concerns about the research nurse role, Shelagh argued that if it had worked properly it could have given her more intellectual stimulation and motivation to implement change on the ward – research for her essentially had to have a clinical base.

Achievements and challenges

There were many benefits evident of having two people in the one post. In essence they included the ability to share the responsibilities for a difficult and stressful job with a colleague, the strength of being able to utilize their different skills, the chance to learn from one's partner, and the opportunity it gave to demonstrate collegial approaches to such activities as planning and goal setting. Both agreed that an important aim and, indeed, outcome was the setting up of a ward which was essentially 'a learning organization' – for patients (through an emphasis on patient education and health promotion), for trained staff (through their empowerment and development of autonomy), for students and also for the partners themselves.

It was obviously important to have a shared vision, albeit with different priorities, agreed ways of working and inclinations that were taken into account. The motivation to bring together their collective skills and 'make the job share work' was also vital.

Nevertheless, the experience had its disappointments and challenges too. For example, before Shelagh came she saw the development of primary nursing as a main aim. However, she soon realized that this was not something that you could do specifically. Developments took place as knowledge grew, and this along with changing the beliefs had to be the focus over and above the establishment of structures for primary nursing (Heslop and Sparrow, 1991). Nevertheless, the processes involved were sometimes slow and painful, and the pace of change could be frustrating.

Further there were the tensions of combining a clinical specialist role, especially for Shelagh, and getting the most appropriate model for a management role. Shelagh had to acknowledge that whilst she thrived as an advanced nurse practitioner (the primary nurse *par excellence* referred to above) who drew constantly on research and challenged her own as well as others' practice, when it came to certain aspects of management she was far less happy. This necessitated careful planning with Angela as to who should take responsibility for what. Indeed, Angela considered subsequently that the situation might have been ameliorated earlier if they had moved more quickly to the current system in place, whereby the staff nurses share more of the management role.

It was unfortunate that Shelagh's research nurse role was not set up well and tended not to complement her job share role, though her research orientation clearly had benefits for her clinical work. But perhaps the most difficult and stressful constraints, and certainly the ones that in discussion Angela and Shelagh returned to again and again were those to do with the organization. These included the fact that the job share post and their other responsibilities did not fit neatly into the traditional hierarchy, which some found difficult to understand and accept. Second, and related to this, the expectations of others did not always meet with the beliefs and the visions of the two and this at times caused friction. Third, the ward tended to be scapegoated – both positively and negatively – because it was seen as 'unusual'. On occasions it was held up as a model to follow, but at other times it was viewed as 'a thorn in the flesh'. Finally, far from being immune from resource restrictions, quality could not always be maintained which is a source of concern for practitioners who are striving not just to maintain the *status quo* but for improved patient care.

Conclusion

This story illustrates that Angela and Shelagh not only believed in the advantages of two nurses at a senior level combining forces in the management and development of a clinical setting, but also that they saw the critical job as comprising management, practice, education *and* research. In this respect they were operating in a unified role, but one where the component parts were shared amongst two people with mutually supporting skills, expertise and interests. They would argue that they did have the requisite authority to manage and to change the clinical environment, though they were at times hampered by organizational constraints.

In addition, their other roles fed into the job share, perhaps more successfully, or certainly less problematically in Angela's case. Through the structure of their various roles, by the ways in which they went about their work, and as shown through their attitudes and beliefs, they were constantly attempting to bring theory and practice together, with the focus for this being very much the practice domain.

Postscript

Shelagh has left the job share, but since her departure, and the change to Angela's role, the management structure has altered. In summary, the primary nurses have taken on more responsibility, the ward sister post is filled with a full-time nurse, and two more of the ward staff have joint appointments between the ward and the respiratory nursing service. (This now comprises five people including a district nurse and a health visitor who are sharing one half-time post.) After two experiences of job sharing, Angela, whilst sanguine about the constraints, still believes in both the theory and practice of job sharing.

Shelagh is now a lecturer practitioner in research (she both facilitates and does research) in another health authority, and Angela is the Senior Nurse for the Nursing Development Unit which emanated from the medical ward, and continues to be a half-time respiratory health worker

References

Heslop, A. P. and Bagnall, P. (1988) A study to evaluate the intervention of a nurse visiting patients with disabling chest disease in the community. *Journal of Advanced Nursing*, **13**, 71–77

Heslop, A. P. and Sparrow, S. (1991) Consensus – a basis for introducing primary nursing into an acute respirology ward. In *Primary Nursing in Perspective* (eds S. Ersser and E. Tutton). Scutari Press, London

Lathlean, J. (1987) *Job Sharing a Ward Sister's Post*. Ashdale Press, Peterborough

Lempp, H. and Heslop, A. P. (1987) Pioneering spirit. *Senior Nurse*, **7**(2), 24–26

Rosser, R., Denford, J., Heslop, A., Kingston, W., Macklin, D. and Minty, K. (1983) Breathlessness and psychiatric morbidity in chronic bronchitis and emphysema: a study of psychotherapeutic management. *Psychological Medicine*, **13**, 93–110

Sparrow, S. (1986) Primary nursing. *Nursing Practice*, **1**, 142–148

11

Nursing Development Units

Steve Wright

Introduction

'You may have learned it like that in the classroom – but that's not
how it's done on the wards'. This comment from an early report
(Bell, 1950) indicates that the belief in the difference between
what nurses are taught in theory and what happens in the reality of
practice is not new. Given that the tension between theory and
practice appears to cause many problems for nursing, a number of
approaches have been attempted in an effort to reduce it. As
already described in Chapter 2, efforts have been made to involve
clinical staff in the activities of the school of nursing, teachers have
been encouraged to spend some of their time in nursing practice,
and roles such as clinical teachers, joint appointments and lecturer
practitioners have been created.

To some extent, the evolution of Nursing Development Units
(NDUs) is a response to this underlying problem. There are
indeed other reasons for their emergence, but their attemps to
bring people and ideas together, to provide a climate where
learning and innovation flourish, and to provide settings where
the goals of education can be coterminous with those of practice,
are evidence of their potential contribution to narrowing the
gap between the theory and practice of nursing. Thus NDUs are
not a panacea to resolve the theory and practice conflict, but they
do offer one direction amongst a range of others to help reduce it.
In addition, it needs to be noted that they are not simply places
where nursing theory, as taught in the academic department,
is transferred in some ideal way into the practice setting. The

relationship between the two settings is not so simplistic or linear. The NDU possesses its own energy, and may itself be producing ideas and innovations. It therefore provides a setting where the generation of nursing theory is driven by developments in practice. The traditional model of theory being created and expanded in one setting, which then transfers it, or passes it down to the practice setting, is overly simplistic. In exploring the concept of the NDU, this chapter will put forward the idea that they set a new dynamic in the traditional framework, and that theory generation and application becomes a function of the practice setting itself.

What is a Nursing Development Unit?

The concept of the NDU is not new. Hall (1969) has described the work and purpose of the Loeb Centre in New York and Christman (1976) an innovative programme at Rush University in Chicago. In the United Kingdom the Royal Marsden Hospital built a reputation for advancements in nursing practice during the 1970s and the professorial unit in Manchester was the first of its kind in England (McFarlane and Castledine, 1982). The title 'Nursing Development Unit' seems to have been applied initially in the United Kingdom to a small community hospital in Burford, Oxfordshire (Pearson, 1988) in the early 1980s and to a large care of the elderly unit in Tameside Health Authority, Ashton-under-Lyne (Wright, 1986). Recent support from the King's Fund Centre has produced a gathering momentum in the foundation of NDUs in the United Kingdom.

Many other settings appear to be pursuing similar goals to NDUs and achieving similar results, although they have not adopted the formal title. What binds them all together in a common approach is not a unified name or a focus on one particular nursing activity. Rather, the totality of their aims, innovations and outcomes is what marks them out as different. Thus each one is concerned not so much with the development of one particular element of nursing but with many, and often simultaneously. There are many places where nurses have introduced a new idea, for example primary nursing. While this illustrates a willingness to change nursing practice, it does not necessarily signify that they are 'Nursing Development Units' as such.

NDUs are therefore settings where change in nursing is an accepted, not unusual, norm of the organization. They enable nursing theory to be put into practice, by providing a setting where learning and ideas flourish and can be applied. At the same time, they are also in the business of generating theory. By testing out new approaches to care, they can provide a feedback system into the body of nursing knowledge; a two-way exchange system which provides a dynamic process for the accumulation and expansion of nursing knowledge and skills.

A clinical nurse specialist from an NDU describes its special contribution as follows:

> I think some of the vistors to the unit wonder just what it is that makes this unit different. I don't find it particularly easy to explain, but it seems that it's not so much a matter of one or two things but of many. For example, on this small unit we have:
>
> - developed a nursing philosophy, model and objectives;
> - changed the management style;
> - introduced a quality assurance programme;
> - developed new clinical specialist roles;
> - written our own nursing standards;
> - devised a standards evaluation package;
> - introduced a comprehensive staff development programme;
> - implemented primary nursing;
> - changed the skill mix of staff;
> - given patients access to their nursing notes;
> - introduced massage and aromatherapy;
> - introduced reminiscence and pet therapy;
> - set up our own nursing beds;
> - gone out of uniform;
> - started taking meals with patients;
> - begun a self medication programme;
> - set up our own nursing library;
> - set up a variety of research projects;
> - created our own fund to support nursing developments;
> - devised information books for patients.

These are just a few of our activities and we seem to be constantly adding more. For us, the NDU provides the umbrella under which an enormous range of nursing activity is under way.

Thus, as Salvage (1989) points out, 'these units which offer the usual range of services to patients as well as some promising innovations, aim to become centres of nursing excellence in their hospital, neighbourhood or health authority. They launch and evaluate experiments in good practice, supported by sound education, management and research. Close relationships with other health authority staff are also fostered'. She goes on to suggest that 'the type of setting and the work undertaken varies according to local needs and initiatives, but all NDUs share a commitment to practicing the best possible standards of nursing, and to sharing with others the insights gained through close scrutiny of their work' (Salvage, 1989). Such units therefore cover the work of health visitors, community nurses, midwives, mental health nurses and others as well as general hospital nurses.

Although the term Nursing Development Unit has become widely accepted because it emphasizes the development of both nurses and nursing, it is not and has no need to be a strictly and universally applied label. It provides a generic term enabling many different units to apply their own name, with which they feel most comfortable. The NDU is a part of any health organization which is specifically and explicitly committed to the development of nurses and nursing practice. Nurses remain the biggest single group of professional employees in health care. In both hospital and community they are one of the few occupations to provide a round-the-clock service. As such, what nurses do and how well they do it, are probably the biggest single factors which directly affect the quality of care the patient or client receives. The relationship between the existence of NDUs and the provision of a nursing service is a simple equation – developing nurses leads to improvements in the quality of their knowledge and skills, which in turn improves the care given to the user of the service.

Pearson (1983) provides the foundations for much current thinking about NDUs. He lays great emphasis on the use of change theory to help develop nursing. Wright (1989a) posits that NDUs accept change as 'a way of life' and agrees that the purposeful application of change theory to nursing practice is an essential component of its work. He suggests that a number of other key features serve to identify the nature of an NDU:

1   It is managed directly by nurses – controlling its own budget, appointment of staff and so on, and its place within the structure of the organization is clearly defined.
2   The aims, objectives and activities are officially acknowledged and sanctioned by the authority/management.
3   The aims and objectives are fully documented, and agreed and reviewed by its nursing staff.
4   Nursing practice is based on an explicit model of care, developed by and continuing to develop with, the clinical nurses.
5   It operates on the basis of an agreed philosophy of care, espousing patient-centred practice and the value of nursing as a therapeutic art and science.
6   The organization of care is based on methods which promote accountability, autonomy, comprehensiveness and continuity of practice by individual nurses within the multidisciplinary team. Methods such as primary nursing therefore tend to be preferred.
7   Quality assurance methods are in operation which involve nurses, other members of the multidisciplinary team, other carers and relatives/visitors, and patients or clients. This forms part of an overall evaluation process to measure the success of the unit as a whole.
8   The managerial style of the unit promotes maximum nursing involvement in decision-making at all levels, and facilitates a climate of innovation and development.
9   It supports and encourages the development of specialist knowledge and practice and specialist roles in nursing.
10   Staff development opportunities are open to all, available on site and demand-led by clinical nursing staff.
11   It works with the school of nursing and other educational establishments to support research and education, and to develop harmony between theory and practice.
12   It raises and uses funds to help nursing staff with professional development, organizes peer-support groups and committees to stimulate dissemination of knowledge and further innovation. It actively seeks to publish and share its work with others.

An enrolled/associate nurse working on an NDU describes the implications of the change:

I've been here for 15 years, 5 years longer than the NDU itself. The place has changed out of all recognition in that time, and I think the care has got much better. The staff seem happier at their work. In that sense the atmosphere has been completely transformed. Before, it was a typical geriatric unit, we felt we were the bottom of the pile in the hospital. Now I think it would be true to say that we see ourselves as the top, we did it, we made the changes, and now other people look to us for ideas. I feel proud to be part of that, and I get a lot of satisfaction from feeling that care of the elderly is at last recognised as something special.

Whilst not being the only means of producing change in nursing, or of producing a setting which meets the needs of those who are learning about nursing, NDUs do appear to offer one significant way forward. Their emphasis is on attaining high-quality patient-centred practice, of promoting innovation, of stimulating a spirit of enquiry – all of these are central to creating a climate for change. In so doing they can develop a culture of nursing which perceives the gap between theory and practice not as a source of conflict or despair, but as a dynamic border worthy of exploration.

The Nursing Development Unit and the learning climate

As Bendall (1975) has pointed out, one of the fundamental mistakes of nursing has been to 'seperate those who teach from those who practice', a phenomenon which has accentuated the gap between theory and practice. Efforts to rectify this have sought to develop roles in which teachers can also be practitioners, as in the case of joint appointments. Indeed, Wilkinson (1983) has described the creation of a joint appointment not only to narrow the gap between theory and practice in her setting, but also to act as a change agent in the building of an NDU. Because they are founded in practice, NDUs are based in the service setting, although they must have the support of the education sector.

Traditionally, the service side of the organization of nursing has often been accused of neglecting the development of nurses. With the education system separate from the system which provides the nursing service (in terms of organization, funding and so on) there may be some truth in the argument that the service side has tended to abrogate its responsibilities for staff development to the school or college of nursing. Thus a false ditchotomy emerged in nursing where the school was there to do the teaching while the management side got on with the business of providing patient care. The latter is such a dominant priority that developing nursing and nurses can often fall into second place, especially in times of restriction upon resources. When hospital budgets are hard pressed, for example, one of the first cutbacks may be in the funding and time allocated to staff education. If NDUs have been successful, it has been in demonstrating that the service side of nursing has an equal part to play in the development of its staff. This should be seen not as a luxurious provision, but as an essential part of the organization's goal of equal and parallel importance to the provision of its services to patients or clients.

The aforementioned clinical nurse specialist elaborates this point:

> At one time, I think there was a perception that nursing theory was something to be taught in the school, and was then expected to happen in the service side. If it didn't then you would be threatened with the big stick of a visit from the ENB! I think we now see things from a different perspective. The practice side might be the place where we take the nursing model being taught by the school, but we have to apply it and use it in our own way. Similarly, things that we do feed back into the education sector to be added to the nursing theory that is being taught there.
>
> A lot of our activities have also been written and published, so in that sense we can also show how new theory can be created in practice, and then added to a wider sphere of nursing. For example, students might learn about the theory of primary nursing in the college of nursing, and here they can see how to apply it in practice. Similarly, we might experiment with new ideas, for example, trying out some of the complementary therapies and evaluating and researching their effects. This in turn goes back into the school curriculum or gets published and debated, and perhaps experimented with on a broader scale. In that way I think it could be said that the nursing practice setting is making nursing theory too, and adding to the whole body of knowledge about nursing.

And the comments of a nursing auxiliary show that it is not only the trained and more experienced staff who benefit:

I did the care assistants' course. It lasted about two months, part time, I did not have to pay. You know, it was the first time since I came here that I felt 'this is something for me'. I really enjoyed it, I used to look forward to the group meeting every week. I felt more like part of the team; like I was getting something, like I was learning too. You hear about these sort of ideas [Nursing Development Units] and I thought, it will be the usual way, something for the qualified staff; nothing to do with me. Like most of us [nursing auxiliaries] I thought it would not affect me, except to make my work harder while all the trained staff went off on study days. But we all had something and there's lots of different ways, not just courses. But I can't tell you how proud I was when I finished my course. I got a certificate, presented by the Manager. My husband was there. I felt so proud, me for the first time in my life I had something that said I was not thick and had achieved something!!

Orton (1980) clearly demonstrates that it is possible to identify the elements which constitute a positive nursing climate. Two key factors are the management style and the team spirit which help nurses feel that they are able to ask questions, to suggest ideas and to use initiative, without fear of recrimination. A third important factor in the climate is that nurses feel able to deliver care in a way which is patient-centred and which is carried out as they have learned that it should be. Other studies (e.g. McLure *et al.*, 1983; Price Waterhouse, 1988) support the view that where these conditions are not being met, then there is likely to be a high level of dissatisfaction among nurses. This in turn leads to failure to achieve quality care, high staff sickness, absenteeism and leaving rates, and a poor record of staff retention. The following comments of an assistant general manager of a unit with an NDU illustrates this point:

I'm wary of suggesting that there is a direct causal link, and saying that because of this, then this happened. In fact, I think it would be impossible to pin it down to any one factor. However, in the past ten years we've seen the attrition rate of staff fall from 56% to less than 1% now. From the evaluations we've conducted, both among staff who have left and those who are here, it seems that the provision of a development programme, together with an opportunity to be creative in nursing practice, is what keeps people here. This aspect alone makes it worthwhile from a management point of view. Getting rid of a nursing recruitment and retention problem is a major achievement in any managers' objectives.

Nursing theory tends to promote the value of patient-centred practice, and this is reinforced in teaching offered in schools and colleges of nursing (Bendall, 1975; Henderson, 1980; Royal College of Nursing, 1985; United Kingdom Central Council, 1986). When the practice setting fails to live up to these expectations, then the implications for the recruitment and retention of nurses are profound. It has been strongly argued that the managers of nursing can ill afford to ignore these arguments, and that contributing to the development of staff is as much a part of the service sector as the educational one. This is especially so in the light of demographic trends reducing the available pool of potential recruits to nursing, exacerbated by the expansion of job opportunities in other, perhaps less demanding occupations, especially for women (Beardshaw and Robinson, 1990). It seems that it is as important for an organization to invest in its nursing staff, through effective programmes of development and facilitating a patient-centred climate, as it is to invest in new equipment or services. As Beardshaw and Robinson (1990) state, 'nursing shortages together with new approaches to nursing work should contribute to a substantial re-evaluation of nurses' actual and potential contribution to health care in the 1990s . . . it will be important for managers and other policy makers outside nursing itself to understand and support nurses' efforts to improve their contribution to the British health services'.

If the theory and teaching of nursing espouses a patient-centred view of practice, then clearly they share common goals with the work of NDUs, for it is these which seek to put such theory into practice. By providing the 'clinical laboratory' (Infante, 1985), they offer a setting in which learning and innovation in nursing can be practised safely from both the nurse's and the patient's and client's perspective. It is possible to achieve harmony between the aspirations and ideals of education and theory, and the needs and demands of the service.

In providing a setting where there is a spirit of enquiry and learning, where both patients or clients and nurses can have their individual needs met, the NDU seems to offer an important way forward for nursing. This is supported by the views of a third-year student nurse allocated to a ward in a Nursing Development Unit:

> I worked here during my first allocation eighteen months ago, and I asked to come back here in the management module in the run up to my finals. I've found this to be the most satisfying experience of all my training, and I think all of my group feel the same. I felt I was treated like an adult here, I could ask questions and not be made to feel like an idiot. I think it's the place, most of all where I've found that what they told me about in school really does happen on the wards. I get treated as an individual here, and so do the patients. I'm hoping to come and work here when I qualify.

In fulfilling the application of theory and ideals to practice, they also seem able to meet the cost-effective goals of the nursing service organization for high quality care, given by well motivated and well educated staff.

Theory into practice – theory from practice

The relationship between NDUs and nursing theory is neither one way nor linear. The traditional view of nursing theory being taught in the classroom and then carried into practice by the student is too limited. In developing practice and sharing their insights, it is possible for practitioners to generate new theory and to illuminate the astonishing richness, variety and complexity of their work. Benner's (1984) work has helped to reinforce the view that each individual nurse builds up a highly intricate body of knowledge and skills in the transition 'from novice to expert'. Benner has illustrated that nurses use an immense range of theory in their practice. Yet this often goes unrecognized, not least by practitioners themselves as their nursing thoughts and actions seem to emerge automatically in a smooth flow of nursing care. A consultant nurse, in speaking about early nursing experiences, reflected this saying:

> I remember very well one nurse who probably influenced my practice more than any other. She was a sister in charge of a surgical ward, and I was a first year student. I can only describe watching her work as awe-inspiring. She never seemed to bustle or hurry, yet she seemed to get through twice as much work as everybody else.

Her nursing care seemed faultlessly organised and appeared to flow smoothly and effortlessly. When she bed-bathed a patient, he would seem comfortable throughout, and look completely renewed and refreshed afterwards. By contrast, I seemed to take twice as long, and I felt like the whole procedure was a struggle, for both the patient and myself. By the time I'd finished he would look like he'd been 'dragged through a hedge backwards', that's the only way I can described it. I used to feel overwhelmed by what I had to learn and thought that I would never be able to nurse with such skill, with such art, as this woman. I don't think she ever gave me a tutorial or took me to demonstrate a procedure, but I learned so much just by 'being with' her.

It is possible for nurses to take theory with them into practice. For example, they may learn about a particular nursing model and seek to apply it to their situation by using the framework it provides to plan patient care. As a primary nurse observed:

I'd read quite a lot of the nurse theorists work, and some I find difficult to comprehend, especially Martha Rogers. Then I found a link while learning and practising Therapeutic Touch. Rodgers provided a theoretical basis for the study I am doing with patients. Suddenly I find a theory that had seemed remote and incomprehensible being very relevant to my unit.

However they may notice weaknesses or limitations, and seek to modify or develop theory for themselves, and then test it out to see if their ideas work. Similarly practitioners may have an idea, and simply try it out. In so doing, they may be adding to existing theory or may begin the development of new ones. Pearson *et al.* (1988), for example, saw the possibility of developing 'nursing beds' – nurses being in control of the admission, care and discharge of patients for whom nursing was the principal therapy. The project was evaluated and results proved highly positive. Nurses in another unit sought to try out the use of photographs to identify patients, instead of using identity bands, and developed a self-medication scheme to test the possibility of improving patient compliance after discharge (Swiatczak and Williams, 1991). These examples illustrate that dealing with nursing theory is not the exclusive province of the person who only theorizes, nor is theory only concerned with the grand issues or matters related to the 'meaning of life'. In addition, nursing theory is part of a rich interchange between theorizing and practising. The two are rarely separate entities, frequently their boundaries are muddied and blurred. The following comment from an associate nurse illustrates this:

> I helped with the project to look at the use of staff uniforms. We found a lot of opinion on this subject, but not much clear evidence. We had various trials and looked at what patients, staff and doctors thought. A lot of our theories and expectations weren't met. We expected the staff in the acute wards to be very pro-uniform, but after the trial, the majority had changed their views. It also shed a lot of light on what patients expect, and how existing uniforms are hopelessly non-functional. There's more research being done, and the policy on uniforms is now under wholesale review.

Nursing Development Units – the future

Though the general notion of NDUs is not new, their formal evolution and explicit definition is a relatively recent event. While some settings have demonstrated the attributes of those units which might fall within the category of the modern day NDU, it has to be said that most nurses have yet to experience the benefits of their approach. Huge areas of nursing remain locked within the *status quo*. However, if the current nursing literature is any indicator, then in recent years, nursing may be said to have experienced a veritable explosion of innovation and change. A result of this is the expansion of the number of NDUs. Four were created with assistance from the King's Fund Centre in 1989 (Brighton, Camberwell, Weymouth and Southport) and a government grant is supporting another thirty. Further support, by assisting with networking and providing small grants, has enabled continuous expansion to take place. To date, several hundred throughout the United Kingdom have now emerged. In addition, a glance through the nursing press reveals that nurses are involved in a huge range of innovations across the spectrum of nursing, whether this is organized under the aegis of an NDU or not. The King's Fund Centre has initiated an extensive programme of evaluation, and meanwhile, early results suggest that positive benefits accrue from them (Pearson *et al.*, 1988; Wright, 1989b; Turner Shaw and Bosanquet, 1993; Black, 1993).

Nevertheless, an Assistant General Manager sounds a word of caution:

> NDUs have a role to play in developing the practical awareness of nurses, as well as of their practice. That is to say, more nurses need to know how the system ticks, how to achieve their goals, and to preserve what they achieve. The health service is a volatile place, many changes are under way. Nothing is guaranteed or certain. Developing nursing might seem to be a 'good thing', with such obvious benefits for all. But there is no guarantee an NDU will survive any more than any other part of the service – look at Beeson Ward. Nurses have to be constantly on the alert, ready to respond and able to produce irrefutable arguments for developing nursing.

Indeed progress has been marred by setbacks. A major example, referred to above, was the closure of the second NDU on Beeson ward in Oxford in the late 1980s. A principal factor in its demise was the reassertion of medical power over an embryonic nursing unit. It closure was greeted with a furore in nursing circles (Naish, 1989) and led at least to a commitment by the health authority to estabish nursing beds elsewhere. However, the events provide a salutary reminder to nurses that their goals are not always shared by others, and that more powerful groups may exert an influence out of all proportion to their numbers or contribution to health care. Vaughan and Pillmoor (1989) remark that 'in reality the group with the greatest power is likely to make the greatest impact when competing for resources. The imbalance which can occur as a result is not always in the interest of the service'. A primary nurse talks about this issue of power, saying:

> I've changed a lot myself. I know more about nursing and more about me – the self awareness course was part of that. That's another way the NDU can be tested. It can be amusing, and sometimes difficult, when you see people's responses, especially those who think they know best. Sometimes, you feel it quite strongly from them – especially some doctors or managers or nurse teachers. I mean, you can see it on their faces. 'Who is this little staff nurse daring to stand up to me and have ideas of her own'. The power – relationship shifts, and you can tell that not everyone, especially those who are used to being in control, like it.

Change in nursing has rarely exhibited a smooth path, and the traditional view that nursing has continued to progress inexorably from the dark ages to modernity seems somewhat naive. In reality, nursing has often lurched from one event to another, sometimes forwards, sometimes in reverse. The history of change in nursing has been more one of volatility and unpredictability rather than smooth transition. Whether NDUs will prove an exception to this rule remains to be seen.

If NDUs continue to be successful in contributing to the expansion of the body of knowledge of nursing, then they will have played their part in enabling nursing to take up its full role within the multidisciplinary team. As Vaughan and Pillmoor (1989) indicate, 'the reality of a need to review our current practice must be faced : . . . the body of knowledge on which practice is based must be sound . . . the relationship between nurse and patient must move from one of directorship to one of partnership . . . the organisation in which nursing works must be transformed to move from a tight hierarchy to a structure which fosters growth'. NDUs are an approach to achieve these goals. In time, if they succeed, then perhaps the label will be irrelevant, for every nursing setting will be a Nursing Development Unit.

Conclusion

NDUs aim to provide the milieu in which the application, testing and generation of nursing theory can take place. They offer nursing one more tool by which change and innovation can supersede stagnation and powerlessness. They aim to provide a climate which fosters creativity, enquiry and patient-centred practice. In so doing they form part of a movement in nursing which Salvage (1990) has described as the 'new nursing' – the evolution, some might say a return to certain values in nursing which espouse the essential worth and complexity of nursing practice. Roles tend to be established which combine the managerial, teaching, research and practice elements of nursing in an effort to produce greater congruence between the theory and practice of nursing. This may include the creation of joint appointments, clinical specialist or nursing consultant roles.

NDUs tend to work with nursing educational establishments, not only to take mutual advantage of each others activities, but also pursue the common goals which both share. The aim of a high quality nursing service is intimately bound up with the development of nursing and nurses. Contributing to both is a proper investment by both the education and service sectors of nursing. They are but one option for nursing to achieve its aspirations and ideals; they are not the panacea to nursing's ills. However, by placing the development of nursing practice firmly on the agenda, by demonstrating that nursing practice provides the opportunity to apply theory to and grow in practice, they give nurses a stepping stone into the future.

References

Beardshaw, V. and Robinson, R. (1990) *New for Old – Prospects for Nursing in the 1990s.* King's Fund Research Report No. 8, King Edward's Hospital Fund for London

Bell, G.M. (1950) Report of the Annual General Meeting of the ward and departmental sisters' section of the Royal College of Nursing. *Nursing Times*, **46**(29), 3–4

Bendall, E. (1975) *So You Passed, Nurse.* Royal College of Nursing, London

Benner, P. (1984) *From Novice to Expert: Excellence and Power in Clinical Nursing Practice.* Addison-Wesley, California

Black, M. (1993) *The Growth of Tameside Nursing Development Unit.* King's Fund Centre, London

Christman, L. (1976) Educational standards versus professsional performance. In *Current Perspectives on Nursing Education* (ed. J. A. Williamson), C. V. Mosby, St Louis

Hall, L. E. (1969) The Loeb Centre for Nursing and Rehabilitation. *International Journal of Nursing Studies*, **6**, 81–95.

Henderson, V. (1980) Preserving the essence of nursing in a technological age. *Journal of Advanced Nursing*, 5, 245–260.

Infante, M. S. (1985) *The Clinical Laboratory in Nursing Education.* Wiley, Chichester

McFarlane, J. L. and Castledine, G. (1982) *A Guide to the Practice of Nursing Using the Nursing Process.* C. V. Mosby, London

McLure, M. L., Poulin, M. A., Sovie, M. D. and Wandelt, M. A. (1983) *Magnet Hospitals – Attraction and Retention of Professional Nurses.* American Academy of Nursing, Kansas City

Naish, J. (1989) Picking up the pieces. *Nursing Standard*, **3**(25), 13

Orton, H. (1980) *The Ward Learning Climate.* Royal College of Nursing, London

Pearson, A. (1983) *The Clinical Nursing Unit.* Heinemann, London

Pearson, A. (1988) (ed) *Primary Nursing: Nursing in the Burford and Oxford Development Units.* Croom Helm, London

Pearson, A., Durand, I. and Punton, S. (1988) *Therapeutic Nursing: An Evaluation of an Experimental Nursing Unit in the British National Health Service.* Burford and Oxford Nursing Development Unit, Oxford

Price Waterhouse (1988) *Nurse Retention and Recruitment.* Price Waterhouse, London

Royal College of Nursing (1985) *The Education of Nurses: A New Dispensation. Commission on Nursing Education* (Chairman: Judge). Royal College of Nursing, London

Salvage, J. (1989) Nursing Developments. *Nursing Standard*, 3 (22), 25

Salvage, J. (1990) The theory and practice of the new nursing. *Nursing Times*, 86 (4), 42–45

Swiatczak, L. and Williams, K. (1991) Prescription for change. *Nursing the Elderly*, 3 (1), 26–27

Turner Shaw, J. and Bosanquet, R. (1993) *Nursing Development Units: A Way to Develop Nurses and Nursing.* King's Fund Centre, London

United Kingdom Central Council For Nursing Midwifery and Health Visiting (1986) *Project 2000: A New Preparation for Practice.* UKCC, London

Vaughan, B. and Pillmoor, M. (1989) *Managing Nursing Work.* Scutari Press, London

Wilkinson, K. E. (1983) Blueprint for a joint appointment. *Nursing Times*, 79 (42), 29–30

Wright, S. G. (1986) *Building and Using a Model of Nursing.* Edward Arnold, London

Wright, S. G. (1989a) Defining the Nursing Development Unit. *Nursing Standard*, 4 (7), 29–31

Wright, S. G. (1989b) *Changing Nursing Practice.* Edward Arnold, London

12

The lessons learnt

Barbara Vaughan

Introduction

There is no doubt that seeking ways of unifying theory and practice is a demanding task since inherent in the effort is the need for change. Furthermore the work required will never be complete as new ideas and knowledge emerge, the context in which health care is delivered alters, and the prevailing ideologies which drive society shift. Few would wish to live in a static world, even if there are times when we would like the pace to slow down a little. What is becoming ever more critical, however, is that we gain some control over both the pace and the direction of the changes, planning them proactively with a specific purpose in mind.

Maybe this is one of the most important features which unites the people who have contributed to this book. While they all offer different perspectives, they are also clear about the rationale behind their efforts and the direction they are moving in. Thus, despite the individuality of the varying descriptions it is possible to draw out some themes and ideas which are common throughout.

The value of nursing

There appears to be a fundamental characteristic shared by all who have contributed which relates to an inherent belief in the value of nursing, coupled with a desire to improve the quality of the service which is offered to patients. This underlying link, which holds them all together, brings with it a curiosity about what constitutes good practice alongside efforts to find ways of improving the service which is offered.

Despite this common theme, in terms of a desire to offer better patient care, the angles from which the problem of bringing together theory and practice have been addressed are different. In some instances the developments have been approached directly through initiatives such as NDUs, the exploration of new roles or the introduction of new patterns of work organization. In other cases they have been tackled indirectly through rigorous research to gain insight into the way in which experienced nurses work, personal development initiatives, and changes in priorities of work. But the end point is the same. It goes beyond theorizing from the distance about what may or may not work, to action which has been happening in an attempt to understand or alter the real world of nursing.

Visionaries

A question which this leads to is 'what has motivated these people to bring about change?'. One fundamental principle of successful change management is that those who are involved are clear about the purpose of their efforts (Pearson, 1992). This certainly holds true in the context of this book since all of the contributors went about their work in response to a felt need, albeit at a personal or an organizational level. To some extent a pattern can be seen of concerns about the apparent gap existing between what was happening and what they believed should happen.

Some may describe them as visionaries who have asked questions or seen ways in which the dissonance which such a gap creates can be resolved. They are certainly people who have gained great satisfaction from working with patients but it may be worth speculating whether there are other characteristics which have led them to seek a new order of things. A possible answer could be that they have all undertaken advanced study in the discipline of nursing.

It is only in fairly recent times that there have been opportunities for many nurses to study their own discipline to this level, since a decade ago there were very few chances of studying nursing itself in accredited academic courses as the availability was so sparse. Furthermore, the theoretical literature was limited and nursing research was still in short supply. In consequence very few practitioners or teachers had actually been in a position to explore the underlying theoretical perspectives of their own subject in depth. However, this is no longer the case as in recent times there has been a wealth of new research and literature and the number of graduate and postgraduate courses, and departments has rapidly increased.

While it is difficult to argue for cause and effect it is apparent in this group of nurses, that they all have a firm grasp of nursing from both a theoretical and a practical stance. Thus to some extent, prior to the work described here, they had already started to build bridges between their own personal understanding of nursing and their daily work. It can be speculated that this may be one of the factors which has enabled them to see ways of taking practice initiatives forward in such a creative way.

The joy of nursing

While some effort has been put into alternative ways of helping students to learn about nursing maybe there is a more fundamental issue in these people's backgrounds. This is about finding ways that have allowed experienced practitioners to retain responsibility for practice while developing their careers and extending their own understanding of both theory and practice. Indeed one of the apparent themes in this work is the joy which is gained by people in very diverse roles through the experience of clinical nursing. It is also evident that many of the contributors have kept careful records of the work which they have undertaken, often using journals or reflective diaries (Boud *et al.*, 1985) as a means of unravelling what was happening in their own minds.

In exploring effective practice through analysis of critical incidents, Cahill (1993) has suggested that there are some intrapersonal factors which are experienced by many nurses despite their clinical speciality. She describes one of them as a *transference of energy* which can be both draining and energizing.

On a more personal level Vaughan (1992) has discussed this feeling of energy which was gained for her during the experience of practice while working as a lecturer, which could act as a spur to achieve other work. It would seem that many of the people who explore nursing themselves, whether as teachers, researchers, practitioners or in combined roles, also get this 'buzz' from clinical work which spins off into other aspects, not only of their own lives but also into the lives of those with whom they work.

Thus as they work across boundaries they can take with them the reality of practice which in turn can be fed into decisions which are being made within other aspects of their work. Cox (Chapter 7), for example, talks of the way she can bring her teaching to life by using recent experiences as exemplars. She also describes the influence which her practice has on her research, guiding and informing the questions she asks. Similarly the lecturer practitioners (Chapters 4, 5 and 6) and the job sharers (Chapter 10) have all gained essential credibility in practice and can work with, and understand, the experiences of the students and create realistic and meaningful learning contracts. In expanding the boundaries of their work these nurses appear to theorize on their feet. They have experimented with a new order of things, which has been facilitated by the roles they hold, where traditional frontiers have often been crossed. Even when they have moved into positions which appear at first sight to be less radical, they have taken the opportunity to develop them in such a way as to meet both their own needs and corporate needs. Thus it could be said that practice nurtures them as people while their experiences of practices in turn nurtures other aspects of their work.

Part of a team

From the perspective of these writers the impact of working in new roles is by no means confined to the incumbents themselves. The descriptions which have been given indicate that there is a marked relationship between the development of the clinical leaders fulfilling roles such as lecturer practitioners, practitioner lecturers and NDU leaders, and the development of the people they work with.

These changes seem to have occurred at two levels. First,

through structural alterations, the staff themselves have fuller work roles. For example, FitzGerald (Chapter 4) has outlined the early stages of her work as a lecturer practitioner, emphasizing that the starting point had to be the development of practice and hence the development of the staff. From her work it is apparent that the difficulties of a move from a traditional staff nurse role to working as a primary nurse should not be underestimated, nor the time which is needed to help people to prepare for such transition. This is evident in the work of the job sharers too (Chapter 10). Similarly accepting the responsibility of mentoring (Chapter 6) allows room for staff nurses to develop their skills into the realms of teaching, bringing with it unification at an early stage in their career development. From the quotes that Wright includes (Chapter 11) the change, not just in practice, but in the enjoyment of practice, is evident for the whole team.

There is currently a great deal of talk about empowerment (Salvage, 1992), with arguments that patients cannot be empowered without staff first recognizing and accepting their own authority. One of the underlying themes here appears to be a recognition that in changing the work of one part of a team, there will be an impact on the work of other team members. While some fight shy of such a move there is a counter argument which suggests that expanding the realms of people's authority is actually empowering for them, provided that they are given adequate time to learn new ways, and support while accepting the additional responsibility. Thus a chain can be seen of clinical leaders who, having recognized their own ability and freedom themselves, help others who work with them to act in the same way. In turn, team members themselves can move to a much stronger position to help patients gain power.

Time management

In many of the chapters the demands on time can be seen as a very real difficulty, certainly in the early stages of the work. There do, however, appear to be lessons to be learned from the experiences described here.

First, there is the time that it takes to establish a new role within an organization. Much concern has been expressed about the way in which primary nursing has been introduced so rapidly in some areas with no time for either staff development or an exploration of how the changes will impact on a wider audience, including the patients. Similarly it has been suggested that a two-year period of development is not unreasonable before units can start to work as NDUs (Turner Shaw and Bosanquet, 1993) and Black (1993) describes a five-year period of work prior to the establishment of Tameside as an NDU. Recognition of the time involved in introducing such changes can be seen as a fundamental issue for many of these writers.

With these thoughts in mind it can be speculated that there should be formal recognition of two phases in such processes. There is an initial period of time when considerable energy is needed to learn new ways of doing things. It could be argued that this stage should be differentiated quite clearly from the point at which early development work has been completed and the environment has become more stable again, a pattern similar to Lewin's (1958) well-known process of unfreezing a situation prior to change, movement and then freezing to a more stable position. Support mechanisms, such as additional staffing or external facilitation could be built into the movement stage, not as an ongoing increase in the number of nurses, but as an active planned part of the overall management. Responsibilities could be phased in so that, for example, the lecturer practitioners have a period of protected time for development of the clinical team, prior to taking on the additional work entailed in the student programme or potential NDUs are given time to clarify their purpose before there is an expectation of publicising the outcomes of their efforts.

What can also be seen in the work of these people is that while time is a very real problem they have tackled the situation openly and sought ways of getting the balance right. Several different strategies have been employed. The important issue is that the difficulty has been acknowledged and plans made to redress it. For example, Burns (Chapter 5) saw quite clearly that she could not be a mentor to all the students, and actively helped the staff nurses to develop in order that they could accept some of this work. Similarly Stevens (Chapter 6) knew that there would be different demands in her work at different times of the year and planned what she has called 'phases' where her priorities would change. For Cox (Chapter 7) there was a need to reconsider priorities and be flexible in the way in which she freed time to work clinically, and Sparrow (Chapter 10) moved away from management activities towards clinical work, partly through inclination but also because of the energy and time she was expending unnecessarily in the former, when her partner was more skilled at it.

While there is a serious issue about the size of some of the roles that have been described here, with the inherent risks of role overload, the perspective of the incumbents has not been to reduce the breadth of their authority and responsibilities. Rather it has been one of seeking ways in which they could actively manage their expanding roles and of finding ways of reorganizing things in order to make them realistic within the time frame of a working life.

Support from colleagues

It would appear that there are times when working towards change can be very isolating as well as bringing with it accusations of elitism. For example, the ward run by Heslop and Sparrow (Chapter 10) was often labelled as 'different' and 'special' but not always in a positive sense, and the two were frequently called to defend the unusual nature of their shared post. The need for support from colleagues, both at a personal and an organizational level, becomes critical in such a situation. While this has not been expressed overtly by all the contributors to this book most have expressed some personal anxiety about their ability to achieve what they have set out to do. It is certainly part of the reality of change and there is a need to build in 'safety nets' to ensure that backup is there when it is required.

In a wider context it has been suggested that there is a critical need for new endeavours such as NDUs, lecturer practitioners, or teachers working clinically to find ways of securing themselves within the establishments in which they work (Black, 1993). This was one of the reasons why the lecturer practitioner role was not piloted on a few sites but introduced as the majority role with responsibility for teaching the practice of nursing. In this way it would not be seen as an anomaly, something which was 'different' from everything else, but a 'norm' for local practice. From Cox's description it can be seen how easily misunderstandings can arise, as she was initially seen as the 'expert' from the university and had to work actively to dispel this myth. Similarly an early experience of the joint appointees (Chapter 9) shows how hard they had to work to become accepted by clinical and other colleagues as a source of help and support rather than a threat and this was a very real issue for the job sharers as well (Chapter 10). These things may sound simple but are very important aspects in the overall management of the changes described.

Interestingly, one of the concerns expressed before many of these people took up unified roles of the one kind or another was the potential conflict which could arise out of joint accountability. However, in reality this does not seem to have created a problem. Admittedly strategies were set up to try to minimize the risk of being torn in two directions, such as a three way performance review, involving all parties concerned, frequent planning sessions between the two job sharers, and joint negotiation between the senior nurse and the collegiate lecturer practitioner. Nevertheless, this difficulty does not seem to be the one which has been realized. It could be that in acknowledging that this was a potential area of conflict – as for example experienced by the early joint appointees in the United Kingdom (Wright, 1988) – mechanisms for counter balancing it have been effective. Maybe it also reflects a recognition of the importance of the work that these people are undertaking, and the maturity of their own approach in managing the way in which they work and prioritize for themselves.

Authority for practice

When lecturer practitioners were first envisaged in the UK (Vaughan, 1987) one of the fundamental features was that the authority for managing both practice and education would be vested in one person. In the majority of cases described here that situation has been achieved albeit a demanding position to assume. Similarly in NDU work the authority for practice development is firmly located in the clinical leader and in these circumstances the incumbents have had the freedom to take control of their work from both parties.

However, it is important to point out that models have also been described here where managerial authority has been vested in (or shared with) another person with a collegiate relationship between the two parties concerned. There are both advantages and disadvantages to either model – sole and shared authority – which may need teasing out. In the shared approach it is feasible to negotiate which aspects of work each participant will take the lead in, as well as the nature of the channels of communication, with opportunities for each person to contribute to the other's thinking. Stevens (Chapter 6) for example talks of the critical importance of the work that she and the senior nurse undertook together and the support which they could give one another. However, she also recalls the time when he moved on and there was a need to renegotiate with a new partner the way in which such a sharing could be continued. Similarly, this process of joint planning and negotiation was at the very heart of Heslop's and Sparrow's relationship (Chapter 10). Indeed while there may be less pressure and a more realistic work load in this approach, there is also the need to negotiate very carefully if it is to be successful.

To some extent this potential hazard can also be seen in joint appointee positions, where there could be some confusion for others about who has the authority, since no two people can work in exactly the same way. Furthermore, the joint appointees may also have to clarify where their individual and shared responsibility lies. In Chapter 9 the joint appointees have recalled how important it was for them to choose each other in order that a successful partnership could be formed and should one of those parties leave it is obviously essential that the remaining person has the right to choose who he or she will work with in the future. This was also mirrored in Chapter 10.

A second issue arises in Chapter 9 from the descriptions of the confusion that the students experienced in knowing which of the joint appointees they would be seeing. However in this instance a very proactive solution was found by the participants in changing the pattern of their work so that they could continue to collaborate but respond to student need more effectively. Again it demonstrates the innovative way in which the contributors respond to challenges or difficulties.

Conclusion

Finding ways of intertwining used and espoused theory will continue to be a challenge for all professional practitioners whatever walk of life they work in. However, if our *raison d'etre* is practice then this is something which is worth striving for. Within this book we have recaptured the experiences of some people who have sought to face up to the issue. The approaches that they have taken are by no means exclusive but in sharing their experiences they do offer some guidance to others who may seek to move along similar paths. It is possible to identify key features which recur in many of the chapters (Figure 12.1) and these would need to be addressed in the future as new approaches continue to be developed. With these themes in mind, steps can be taken to manage them purposefully and thus minimize some of the potential hazards.

All the people who have contributed to this book knew that they would be taking risks in moving into new territories, but none of

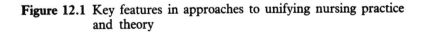

- ☐ A belief in the value of nursing
- ☐ A commitment to the knowledge inherent in practice
- ☐ The freedom to take risks supported by employers
- ☐ A recognition of the time needed to establish new roles
- ☐ The influence of continuing education and the need for development opportunities for all involved
- ☐ An ability to prioritize and not try to be all things to all people
- ☐ An ability to manage time effectively, developing purposeful strategies in response to high demands
- ☐ Team work within a mutually supportive environment
- ☐ The courage to act

Figure 12.1 Key features in approaches to unifying nursing practice and theory

them fled from such responsibility. As Orlando (1987) has said when talking of role expansion or role extension, to some extent our future lies in our own hands. While this may be a frightening reality, truth can be seen in such words, but as long as there are nurses around who can see ways forward and have the courage to put their words into action then the future bodes well for nursing.

References

Black, M. (1993) *The Growth of Tameside Nursing Development Unit.* King's Fund Centre, London

Boud, D., Keogh, R. and Walker, D. (1985) *Reflection: Turning Experience into Learning.* Kogan Page, London

Cahill, M. (1993) *Effective Nursing – An Exploration by Experienced Nurses.* Ashdale Press, Oxford

Lewin, K. (1958) Group decision and social change. In *Readings in Social Psychology* (ed. E. Maccoby). Holt, Rinehart and Winston, New York

Orlando, I. (1987) Nursing in the 21st century. *Journal of Advanced Nursing*, **12** (4), 405–412

Pearson, A. (1992) *Nursing at Burford: A Story of Change.* Scutari Press, London

Salvage, J. (1992) The new nursing: empowering patients or empowering nursing. In *Policy Issues in Nursing* (ed. J. Robinson). Open University, Milton Keynes

Turner Shaw, J. and Bosanquet, R. (1993) *Nursing Development Units: A Way to Develop Nurses and Nursing.* King's Fund Centre, London

Vaughan, B. (1987) Bridging the gap. *Senior Nurse*, **6** (5), 30–31

Vaughan, B. (1990) Knowing that and knowing how: the role of the lecturer practitioner. In *Models for Nursing 2* (eds B. Kershaw and J. Salvage). Scutari Press, London

Vaughan, B. (1992) Exploring the knowledge of nursing practice. *Journal of Clinical Nursing*, **1** (3), 161–166

Wright, S. G. (1988) Joint appointments; handle with care. *Nursing Times*, **84** (1), 32–33

Index